Depre
Immatu.. Romance.

A Constructive Guide to the Causes, Cures, Types, and Secret Inner Psychology of Depression

By Roman Gelperin

Depression and the Immature Romance: A Constructive
Guide to the Causes, Cures, Types, and Secret Inner Psychology of
Depression, by Roman Gelperin

Visit the author's website at: www.RomanGelperin.com

Copyright © 2019 Roman Gelperin

Legal Disclaimer:

ISBN: 9781097897582

Acknowledgements

I'd like to thank my ex-girlfriend, Amirah. In dating me, talking with me, sharing her life story with me, and living with me while I was writing this book, she gave me a new and invaluable secondhand perspective on depression. And I'd like to thank my editor, Ed Levy, for helping me refine some of the book's content.

Table of Contents

Preface

The flash of insight that birthed this book came to me in late 2012, when—in my aspirations to become a psychological therapist (long since abandoned)—I was struggling to crack the puzzle of depression. The condition seemed a bizarre and baffling one to me at the time, and the more I read up on it—absorbing the clinical descriptions of its symptomology in psychiatric manuals; reviewing hundreds of firsthand accounts of it on the psychology and depression forums online; and checking out all the popular psychology books the New York Public Library had on the topic—the more confusing and incomprehensible the subject became. Mainstream psychology, to which I first turned looking for insight, could offer no adequate explanation of this affliction, as it continues to be unable to for the countless individuals currently suffering from depression.

Everything I read, and all the videos I watched on depression, simply didn't go *deep* enough. "Out of the blue," writes Richard O'Connor—psychotherapist, lifelong depressive, and author of *Undoing Depression*, by far the best and most brilliant book currently available on the subject—is "one of the favorite phrases of depressed people." It is an expression of their assumption, and their experience, that their feelings, symptoms, and mood changes come out of nowhere—as random, chaotic events they can't understand or control. But "nothing comes out of the blue," notes Richard O'Connor. And every change in mood or sudden onset of a depressive episode is really caused by a fleeting mental event the depressed person experiences but isn't aware of.

I too, by way of meticulous introspection into the depths of my own mind, had long since discovered this principle: that there is nothing causeless in human psychology. And it was precisely these fleeting, unconscious mental processes underlying depression—the secret inner churnings of the depressed mind—that I looked to un-earth to truly understand it. But where could I possibly acquire this knowledge?

At first, I sought the answers from mainstream, "scientific" psy-chology; but I soon learned that when it came to depression, as with countless other questions about the human psyche, this so-called "science" had cut itself off from precise knowledge of what truly takes place inside the mind—having explicitly banned introspection from among its methods. The books and academic papers I read of this persuasion all had one thing in common: They treated depressed people's minds as if they were black boxes, being allowed to observe their inputs (the depressed people's case histories) and their outputs (their behavior; their symptoms; and even their verbal disclosures about the things that they thought or felt, which were invariably oversimplified, abridged, or disguised versions of what those people were actually thinking and experiencing), but never to peer directly inside of a black box, to empirically examine the inner mechanics that turned its inputs into its outputs. Those pivotal mental pro-cesses, if they were considered at all, were meant to be *inferred* from the physically observable behavior—usually only leading to tentative, superficial, or erroneous theorizing. And detailed introspective de-scriptions, whether cited from an external source or from the au-thor's own inner observations, were entirely left out of this psychological literature.

So, I shifted my focus to autobiographical accounts and mem-oirs. But there too, and chiefly as a result of their "out of the blue" premise, I was faced with the same fundamental problem: These au-thors, practically without exception, treated their own minds as if they were black boxes, describing the circumstances behind their de-pression, the way they acted, and the things they said to the people around them—in short, all the things that would be evident to an outside observer—without delving to any great depth into the pri-vate, intimate details of their mental lives that were available only to themselves.

My last hope, then, was to find an individual who didn't conform to these two trends: A former depressed person, who—in the
course of his illness and recovery—had gained introspective clarity
as to the causes, nature, and cure of his own depression, and pro-
ceeded to write it out as a way to inform others; or maybe a psychotherapist, who had seen dozens of depressed people in his private
practice, and decided to solicit the most in-depth introspective re-
ports he could get from them, and then publish them in a collection.
After extensive searching, however, I arrived at the verdict that such
an exception probably didn't exist; that if an account like it existed,
its contribution to our uncertain understanding of depression would
not have gone unnoticed; and if it existed, but in near total obscurity,
so that no one in the field knew about it, my own chances of finding
it were likewise extremely slim.

I had, it is true, myself experienced a period of depression during my adolescence—after the breakup of my first romantic relationship. But that experience seemed so strange and atypical to me—and
so different from the much more intense, ingrown, convoluted kinds
of depression I was reading about—that I came to view it as an odd-
ity peculiar to myself: as a totally unimportant, idiosyncratic chapter
of my life that I never quite understood or bothered to understand;
and which, above all, had no wider relevance to the general illness of
"depression" that other people so frequently talked about and experienced.

And then, in the course of my research into depression, I read
Freud's *Mourning and Melancholia*. This brief ten-page essay, though
not the introspective account I was looking for, instantly
revolutionized everything I understood, and didn't understand,
about depression. It paralleled my own depressed episode perfectly,
analyzed it ingeniously (and, I must say, very correctly), and showed
it to be *not* some odd irrelevancy peculiar to myself, but in fact a
highly typical case (of at least one kind) of depression. Vivid
memories of that time came rushing back to me, suddenly coherent
in the light of Freud's insights; and I found I was able—with this
reclaimed introspective knowledge, plus my considerable knowledge

of human psychology and emotions—to understand the essence, causes, and cures of depression (or at least this one kind of depression) from personal experience.

That is how this book came about. I saw that now, I was able to give readers the knowledge I searched for but couldn't find: A firsthand, introspective account of what takes place in the mind of a depressed person, and the way this produces his psychological symptoms. In addition, I could fill in the gaps and resolve the confusion in Freud's own theory, using some of my personal insights and observations.

For any reader interested in depression—whether because he suffers from it himself, has a friend or family member who does, or simply out of intellectual curiosity—I trust this book to provide him with an enlightening new understanding, and at a depth of analysis not seen in contemporary psychology, that he will not encounter anywhere else.

Author's Note

Although, in a burst of inspiration, I completed the first manuscript of this book in 2013, I didn't set to revising it to be published until five years later. In working on this revision, I was intent on making my book as well-researched as possible, in contrast to the original manuscript, which drew primarily on my personal experience. During this process, I ended up reading nearly two dozen whole books on depression, as well as countless scientific papers, and for a year-and-a-half even dated a girl with a long history of major depression, childhood trauma, and attempted suicide, all of which shaped and informed this final version.

To my surprise, I found the existing literature on depression much more insightful than I had remembered. Authors like Richard O'Connor, Andrew Solomon, and Aaron Beck wrote highly intelligent, illuminating books that greatly furthered my understanding of depression. A wealth of published experiments, studies, and statistical data on the psychology, biology, and sociology of depression provided me valuable information no introspection can ever discover. Only in one place, however, did I find the kind of extensive, in-depth, introspective account of depression I had been looking for, and which I eventually wrote in this book of my own depression. (All other self-reports, autobiographies, and memoirs proved a severe disappointment: introspective psychology is a lost art.) That was *The Autobiography of John Stuart Mill*, which contains perhaps the most detailed, uncensored, self-critical analysis of the causes, firsthand experience, and psychological cure of one's own depression (although a different type of depression than the one I experienced) in all of literature, and which I gratefully used as an example in this book.

While the first and last parts of this book are heavily based on this new information, I left the core of the book ("Chapter 5: Deconstructing Depression" through "Chapter 9: My Personal Encounter with Depression") largely the way I first wrote it. It's written on two levels: the main line of reasoning (in the body) and elaborations on the underlying psychology (in the footnotes). Both are equally valuable, and are intended to be read in order.

Chapter 1

An Overview of Depression

A human is born with a mind, but no knowledge of how it operates. This knowledge must be discovered or learned, afresh, by each individual. But many don't learn, and some only discover the hard way, that in their minds lies the potential for depression.

The first time a person falls into depression—I mean a pathological, clinical depression—the change that takes place in his feelings, personality, and behavior is an entirely alien one to him. This person is helpless against that seemingly foreign entity exerting so dreadful an influence on his body and mind, unable to consciously control it, or understand why this change has occurred. The person who's fallen in love the first time shares a very similar, although benevolent, experience. (The two are, in fact, frequently related, as we shall see later in the book.)

Understanding the human mind and its hidden potentials is, of course, the main purpose of the science of psychology. Helping people understand their own minds also has great benefits for their psychological health. It helps them rationally deal with, or at least become aware of, the elements of their mind they can't consciously control. Yet up to now, psychologists have been decidedly unable to discover the psychological causes of depression—or to determine what takes place in the mind of a person when he becomes depressed. We will see in this book whether a different approach to psychology, an introspective approach, can help shed some much-needed light on this problem.

But let us take a brief survey of what's currently known about depression to put our topic in its proper context.

Melancholia of the Greeks

Depression is by no means a new or even a newly discovered mental illness. It was first described in the 5th century BC by the ancient Greek physician Hippocrates, who named the condition *melancholia*, based on his theory that it was caused by an excess of (what we now know to be a fictitious) black bile—the Greek word for black being *"melas"* and for bile being *"kholé."*

Today (according to the most recent 2015 statistics), 9.5 percent of American adults will suffer from some form of depression in a given year, and about one in every five Americans will experience this affliction in his or her lifetime. Aside from the debilitating effects it has on one's daily life, depression is especially dangerous because of its tendency to lead to suicide, being responsible for two-thirds of all suicide deaths—slaying over thirty-one thousand people a year in the US alone, and just under half of a million worldwide. This makes depression, by far, the most destructive psychological illness in the world today.

Depression in the DSM

The fourth edition of the Diagnostic and Statistical Manual of Mental Disorders (the DSM-4), which is the definitive bible of American psychiatry, breaks what we commonly call "depression" into three distinct categories of depressive disorder: (1) Major Depressive Disorder, (2) Dysthymic Disorder, and (3) Depressive Disorder Not Otherwise Specified. Yet the actual difference between these three categories, observes Richard O'Connor, is trivial at best.

"The bottom line," he explains, "is that with major depression," you feel the standard depressive symptoms—sadness, confusion, suicidality, guilt, as well as affected sleep, sex life, and appetite—intensely, "and it hits you rather quickly." With dysthymia, "you feel some or all of the same symptoms, but not as intensely, for at least two years." And with Depressive Disorder Not Otherwise Specified, "you feel many of the same symptoms, but not as intensely as in major depression, and not for as long as [in] dysthymia." He further points out the absurdity that, according to the DSM, a person who qualifies for major depression and for dysthymia receives the diagnosis of "double depression."

We should not, of course, take these DSM categories of mental disorder too seriously, at least from a scientific standpoint. These "disorders" are based much more on practical application than scientific insight, since their main objective is helping the psychiatric professional determine which medications to prescribe—as opposed to isolating a distinct psychological phenomenon. The critical symptoms which qualify a person for a DSM disorder also don't grant us much scientific insight. They are only the general, directly observable surface signs of a psychological illness, selected to allow even the least skilled psychologist—basically anybody with eyes, ears, and a questionnaire—to make a diagnosis with very limited information, which can be gathered in a two-hour interview, without probing to any great depth into the patient's internal life. But just for reference, here are the diagnostic criteria from the DSM-4.

Major Depression, Dysthymia, and Depressive Disorder Not Otherwise Specified

According to the DSM-4, to qualify for Major Depressive Disorder, a person has to have at least five of the following nine symptoms—and at least one of the first two has to be present—for a period of two weeks or more:

1.) Depressed mood (feeling sad or empty) for most of the day, nearly every day

2.) Markedly diminished interest or pleasure in all, or almost all, activities most of the day, nearly every day

3.) Significant weight loss or weight gain, or increase or decrease in appetite most of the day, nearly every day

4.) Insomnia (trouble sleeping) or hypersomnia (sleeping excessively) nearly every day

5.) Restlessness or lethargy of movement nearly every day

6.) Fatigue or loss of energy nearly every day

7.) Feelings of worthlessness or excessive or inappropriate guilt nearly every day

8.) Diminished ability to think, or concentrate, or indecisiveness nearly every day

9.) Recurrent thoughts of death (not merely fear of death), ideas of suicide, or an attempt at committing suicide or specific plans to do so

Each two-week or longer period in which these criteria are met, and that is finally interrupted by a period of "remission" in which the criteria aren't met for at least two consecutive months, is called a Major Depressive Episode.

To qualify for Dysthymic Disorder, the symptomatic requirements are a lot laxer. A generally depressed mood, plus at least two of the following six symptoms—"(1) poor appetite or overeating, (2) insomnia or hypersomnia, (3) low energy or fatigue, (4) low self-esteem, (5) poor concentration or difficulty making decisions, [and] (6) feelings of hopelessness"—have to be present for more days than not over a minimum period of two years.

And if the pattern of a person's depression doesn't meet the criteria for either Major Depression or Dysthymia—whether meeting all the symptoms for Dysthymia, but for less than two years; or falling just short of the five of nine symptoms needed for Major Depression; or meeting all of the symptoms for Major Depression frequently, but for brief periods of less than two weeks—the person can then be diagnosed with Depressive Disorder Not Otherwise Specified.

The Three Categories, a Difference in Degree

These three separate categories, along with the concept of "double" depression (in which a person is diagnosed with both Major Depression and Dysthymia), may give some of us the misconception, writes Richard O'Connor, that these are actually three separate diseases, with three "separate disease processes at work." In his view, however, it's all just a matter of degree—with dysthymia being "what people with major depression feel when they get a little better," major depression being "a more severe version of dysthymia," and Depressive Disorder Not Otherwise Specified being "either the early stage of or a slightly milder case of dysthymia."

He cites a study—in which 431 patients were followed for a period of twelve years after they had a Major Depressive Episode—that just about irrefutably proves his point. During those twelve years, these patients only experienced major depression an average 15 percent of the time; they went on to experience dysthymia, however, an additional 27 percent of the time; and they experienced Depressive Disorder Not Otherwise Specified another 17 percent of the time. Those results speak for themselves.

Persistent Depressive Disorder

The latest edition of the DSM—the DSM-5, first released in 2013—has made an important change to these categories of depression, which apparently concedes O'Connor's point. Acknowledging that "major depressive episodes may occur during [the course of dysthymia]," and failing to find any "scientifically meaningful difference" between the "symptoms, family history, or treatment response" of those diagnosed with dysthymia and those diagnosed with chronic depressive disorder (that is, reoccurring episodes of major depression each lasting two weeks or more, and spanning a period of minimum two years), these two categories have been consolidated into one, and together renamed to Persistent Depressive Disorder. This is, I think, an entirely correct amendment, which I will discuss later.

All the other changes to depressive disorders in the DSM-5 are minor or cosmetic, and will be irrelevant to our upcoming investigation.

Chapter 2

Symptoms and Observations

Outside of the DSM, closer analysis and self-reports of the symptoms of depressed people have yielded the following observations:

Self-Descriptions of Depression

Depressed people frequently describe what they experience using the metaphor of darkness—a feeling of descending into darkness, of being enveloped by darkness. Perhaps most commonly, when their moods are somewhat less intense, they will instead describe it as feeling "blue," or "numb," or "down." They also commonly express the feeling of being weighed down, of having to make great efforts to do even the simplest things, and even the tiniest physical or mental exertion becoming a great, tedious hurdle. Depressed people will often speak of a state of blankness, loneliness, becoming invisible, fading into nothingness, being reduced to zero. They also invariably report feelings of pain and anguish and misery. The emotion of sadness, of course, is nearly always also reported.

Alienation from Sense of Self

One striking and very common experience among depressed persons is a loss of their sense of self. William Styron writes in his memoir of depression, Darkness Visible: "A phenomenon that a number of people have noted while in deep depression is the sense of being accompanied by a second self—a wraithlike observer who, not sharing the dementia of his double, is able to watch with dispassionate curiosity as his companion struggles against the oncoming disaster, or decides to embrace it." Others report this same experience: "From being a living person with a distinct personality I began to feel more or less like an outline of that person. . . . [I was] doomed to impersonate a person I now no longer was." "I was acquiring a new and noticeable detachment from myself, an alienation from the person who spoke and acted for me," "like living in a corpse."

An Unstable Identity

The struggle for identity is also a common theme in persons suffering from depression, and many of them report that even before being overtaken by depression, their lives had been filled with torments over who they were, what they were destined for, and what were their true personalities. During depression this seems to become exacerbated, as the depressed person feels that now, more than ever, he has lost the essence of what he is or used to be.

Roots in Childhood

Many depressed persons also report that even before they broke down into total depression, they had for most of their lives felt its presence nipping at their heels. Many say that there was a constant presence of darkness in their lives, even in their childhood, encroaching upon them once in a while and having to be staved off. And it is well documented that most people who become depressed later in life have also had a seriously troubled childhood, often involving sexual abuse or the death of a parent.

External Blankness, Internal Strife

Another very interesting facet of depression is that contrary to depressed people's inert and lethargic outward disposition, their minds are usually engaged in continual rumination and deliberation. They are perpetually recalling negative events and tormenting themselves over self-debasing thoughts. The best description I have found of it is this one, by fiction writer Leslie Dormen: "One of the many things I hate about the word 'depression' is the assumption of blankness attached to it, as if the experience of depression is as absent on the inside as it looks to be from the outside. That is wrong. Depression is a place that teems with nightmarish activity. It's a one-industry town, a psychic megalopolis devoted to a single twenty-four-hour-we-never-close product. You work misery as a teeth-grinding muscle-straining job . . ., proving your shameful failures to yourself over and over again. Depression says you can get blood from a stone, and so that's what you do. Competing voices are an irritating distraction from the work."

Self-Hatred and Absence of Self-Esteem

A very common observation of depressed persons is that they experience strong feelings of worthlessness, guilt, and self-loathing, together with verdicts of self-devaluation. That they invariably exhibit low, or exactly zero, *positive* self-esteem (positive feelings and judgements about the self, which may exist alongside the negative ones, but most often don't in depressed people), is viewed as an outgrowth of this.

Cognitive Biases

Most depressed people have highly prominent and pessimistic cognitive biases about the past, present, and future. Deeply unhappy now, they have a hard time remembering (and are sometimes wholly unable to remember) any time that they experienced happiness, joy, or fun in the past, even if such times had been plentiful. They tend to interpret present events in an extremely negative, distorted fashion: noticing only the negative aspects of some event, but ignoring the positives ("selective abstraction"); drawing sweeping, disparaging conclusions about their self-worth, what other people think of them, and the nature of the world from a single unpleasant occurrence ("overgeneralization"); viewing minor negative events as catastrophes and massive positive events as insignificant ("maximization and minimization"); and making totally unwarranted, harsh judgments about themselves on the basis of neutral or even positive happenings ("arbitrary inference"). Their view of the future is nearly always bleak, hopeless, and entirely empty of any promise of pleasure, happiness, or fulfillment. They're always expecting the worst. Most poignantly, a depressed person usually can't imagine himself ever feeling better, and expects that his misery will last forever, even though—in the vast majority of cases—this turns out not to be true.

An Episodic Affliction

Depression is, in nearly all cases, episodic: with periods of depression giving way to periods of remission, during which the person feels perfectly well again, or at the very least a lot better. About half of all depressive episodes are over within three months, only a fourth last more than a year, and only about three percent last more than a decade. In at least 50 percent of the persons who recover, however, depression does reoccur; and the remission (lasting anywhere from months to years) is followed by another period of depression (which likewise can last for weeks or for years). And the more episodes of depression a person has had, the more likely he'll be to have another one.

Course of the Illness

The most common course of depression seems to be a gradual onset, followed by increasingly worsening symptoms, until the condition finally "bottoms out" and gradually improves to a complete, or at least partial, remission. Occasionally, however, the onset is a sudden one, a full psychological breakdown—as Andrew Solomon described in *The Noonday Demon*—which leaves the person totally incapacitated, and is followed by a gradual improvement. At other times, it's the recovery that is sudden, and the person's depression can dissipate instantly—without any intermediate improvement—within a single minute, or hour, or day (as happened to me).

Immobile Depression and Workaholic Depression

As the intensity of their depression worsens, most people grow increasingly lethargic, unmotivated, and withdrawn, until—in many cases—they become entirely bedridden. In other people, it takes a different, almost opposite, course. Their depression makes them work even harder, and the more it draws in on them, the harder they work (usually at selfless, thankless tasks that don't get them anywhere) to avoid thinking about it—what Richard O'Connor has called "spinning-your-wheels" depression. It's only when they're forced to take some time off, writes Richard O'Connor, that they "really feel their depression for the first time," discovering "that they have no real interests in life, no relationships, no goals."

A Difference Between First and Subsequent Episodes

An individual's very first episode of depression, many therapists observe, will typically have a recognizable event that precipitated it—

some major tragedy in the person's life that he's well aware of and attributes his depression to. (In some cases, this tragedy may be disguised as a massive success, in which the person finally achieves a long-pursued goal, and finds it to be not what he was expecting, after which life begins to seem meaningless.) The second episode, too, will typically have a precipitating event that the person can identify, but it usually isn't as big a tragedy as the first one. The third and subsequent episodes, however, will often have no precipitating event that the person can recognize, or one so minor that it seems insignificant, and descends upon the depressed person, as he thinks, "out of the blue," but which—as a new school of mindfulness psychologists has shown—is really caused by the person's own thought processes (as I will discuss later).

Avoiding their Feelings

Depressed people, some keen observers note, have an aversive relationship to their feelings, frequently avoiding them because they're afraid to be overwhelmed by them. One depressed woman, who commonly shooed her urges to cry away with the chant—"I've got to be strong. It's silly to feel sad"—was, "[on] some level," afraid that "if she ever started crying, she wouldn't be able to stop; that she would cry for the whole world, for things and for people she['d] lost in her life, for her wrong decisions, for her lost children, for her unfulfilled ambitions."

The Vicious Circle

Depression, countless people observe, is self-reinforcing, a disease that causes itself to spiral downward, a "vicious circle," a positive feedback loop.

Depressed people—even while functional—already over-criticize, blame, and hate themselves for each petty negative incident, for a failure to meet some minor goal or expectation, for a slight or perceived character flaw or inadequacy, which only exacerbates their low mood; then depression bowls them over and practically chains them to their beds, causing them to struggle with even the most basic of daily tasks, makes them unmotivated to achieve any goals or fulfill any promises, and renders them helpless, weak, and pathetic besides, for which they blame themselves even harder.

Depressed people are placed in dire need of the assistance of others; they often desperately crave for connection with others, for genuine friendship, for love, for emotional support. They "walk around with a vast hurt inside and long for someone to heal it," writes Richard O'Connor—but their depression makes them withdraw from other people; it often prevents them from asking for help (or even accepting it when it's offered) by making them feel worthless, unlovable, and undeserving of it; it makes them ashamed of those very needs and desires, and so leads to their hiding them like a guilty secret. The more intense their depression becomes, the further they seek to withdraw into solitude; a blanket of indifference isolates them from their friends and relatives, and genuine connection with others becomes all but impossible.

Depressed people's behaviors are self-sabotaging, and their pessimistic beliefs become self-fulfilling prophecies. Their irrational complaints, their constant threats to commit suicide, their regular acts of self-mutilation—not to mention their apparent ungratefulness and indifference to all help—usually appalls and drives away even those closest to them. Their belief in the worst of all worlds— that nothing good can happen to them, that they're bound to fail at anything they do—frequently leads to them not even trying, to giving up before they have started, to not even seeing the opportunities available to them: a kind of "learned helplessness." And the rare times that they do try—and go to a job interview, or a conference, or a date—they usually do so only half-heartedly, noncommittally, expecting the worst, already assuming that they will fail, which usually leads to actual failure.

Most tragically, depression can cause people to make major, life-ruining decisions—like dropping out of school, terminating an important relationship, or taking up drugs—that will have devastating long-term consequences, undermine their future, and drive them even further down into depression. Such is the circular nature of the illness, and the way that, as Andrew Solomon states, "the symptoms of depression [also] cause depression."

Stress and Depression

A close link between stress and depression has been established by countless studies. Stress is our body's so-called "fight or flight" response—a "nonspecific" biological response to any stimulus that upsets our biological equilibrium, and which is (psychologically) experienced as displeasurable. The stress response sets off a cascade of hormones throughout our body, secreting adrenaline, releasing stored glucose into our blood, speeding up our breathing and heart rate, increasing the blood flow to our muscles and brain—and, at the same time, turning off and inhibiting our digestive and reproductive systems—as a way of mobilizing our body to respond immediately to the disturbance. The strength of this response is proportional to the magnitude of the stimulus—the "stressor." And while it is, in general, extremely useful for taking restorative action in the short term, it can cause serious long-term damage (and the deterioration of one's health) if experienced too frequently.

Stressors and Stabilizers

A major depressive episode is often directly set off by an intense stressor—such as divorce, the loss of one's job, a major humiliation (like discovering infidelity in one's partner), a sudden illness or injury, or the death of a good friend, close relative, or spouse. Furthermore, non-depressed people with genuine, ongoing life difficulties (what are often called "long term stressors")—such as economic hardships, an abusive marriage, legal trouble, the illness of a close family member, the delinquency of one's child, and so on—are a lot more likely to develop depression (about twice as likely, according to one study), even in the absence of any major provoking event.

Those people, on the other hand, who have some source of security in their lives, some internal or external stabilizers that help them diffuse, cope with, or resolve stressful situations, are much less vulnerable, and at a much lower risk of developing depression, than those without them. Those external stabilizers that shield against depression include close friends, supportive relatives, and a "good enough" marriage. And the internal stabilizers include vocational skills, social skills, and general survival skills that give one a sense of control over his life, plus the confidence he can make it through trying times—and for which he must also possess the self-esteem backing those skills.

Vulnerable Demographics

Certain segments of the population that live under difficult circumstances also have higher rates of depression. Women, at least across Western societies, have twice the incidence of depression as men. The elderly living in nursing homes are two times as likely to be depressed as those living outside them. The poor have two to three times the rate of depression of the general population. And gay men, especially in environments that discriminate against them, have up to three times the prevalence of depression as their straight counterparts.

Adverse Childhood Experiences

Adverse childhood experiences are especially significant here.
Children who were frequently beaten by a family member (physical abuse)—were raped or sexually taken advantage of by an adult (sexual abuse)—were frequently threatened, insulted, or called derogatory words by one of their parents (emotional abuse)—had their physical, psychological, and emotional needs ignored by their primary caregiver (neglect)—had seen their mother being physically abused (exposure to a battered mother)—lived with someone who abused drugs or alcohol (exposure to household substance abuse)—

lived with somebody with a psychiatric disorder (mental illness in the household)—saw somebody they lived with go to prison (criminal household member)—or went through their parents' divorce, through one of their parents' deaths, or (even more poignantly) through a parent's suicide—all had, according to countless frequently replicated studies, a much higher incidence of depression as adults. Quite notably, the largest effects from these childhood experiences were produced by emotional abuse toward females, being the child of a depressed parent, and living through the suicide of a parent (each of which approximately tripled the incidence of depression)—although the last two were probably confounded by genetic variables.

More importantly, the effects from these "adverse childhood experiences," called ACEs in the scientific literature, compound. Each additional ACE substantially increases one's vulnerability to depression, which makes their effect on people's chance of developing depression dose-dependent (just like with most drugs, the higher the dose, the more potent will be their effect). The statistics are quite imposing. Even after controlling for genetics, a person with five or more ACEs before age eighteen has a 44 percent chance of meeting the diagnostic criteria for major depressive disorder in any given year of his adult life, and a 61 percent chance of doing so at least once in his adulthood. This is compared to an 8.3 percent one-year prevalence, and a 13.5 percent lifetime prevalence, in adults with zero ACEs; and an 18.5 percent one-year prevalence, and 25.8 percent lifetime prevalence, for those who've had only one ACE.

There's also substantial evidence that, at least for many of these ACEs, the earlier in a child's life they occur, the more at risk for depression they tend to make him. "It has now been established," observes Andrew Solomon, "that depressed children usually go on to become depressed adults." But even if those early experiences don't induce depression right then in childhood—and children as young as two or three are fully capable of experiencing depression— these persons remain much more susceptible to the disorder in their adulthood; and when they do experience it, their depressions tend to be much more intense.

The Compound Effect of Stressors

The effects of current life stressors compound too. In one landmark study of adult women living in a working-class suburb of London, only about 1 percent of the women who experienced no acute or long-term stressor over the one-year course of the study went on to develop depression during that year. For women who did experience an acute or long-term stressor, however, this proportion increased to over 10 percent. For women who experienced the stressor *and* lacked any serious social support, the figure doubled to over 20 percent. And for those who experienced the stressor, lacked social support, *and* either went through the death of their mother before age eleven, had three or more children age fourteen or younger (clearly itself a large long-term stressor), or both, their odds of contracting depression quadrupled to nearly 80 percent.

Long-Term Neurological Changes

On top of all that, a major depressive episode is itself an enormously stressful experience extending over a very long period of time. After every such episode, a person's brain undergoes lasting (though not irreversible) changes in its reactivity to stress: It becomes a lot more sensitive to it, setting off a disproportionately huge stress response in the face of only a small strain. It is after a person has had two, or three, or maybe four major depressive episodes, that even a tiny stressor becomes capable of inducing another one.

Anxiety and Other Mental Disorders

Furthermore, these changes in the brain's stress reactivity also affect anxiety reactivity in the same way. Depressed people, especially chronically depressed people, will very often have troubles with anxiety—and many studies, including a massive one by the World Health Organization, have found that 51 to 68 percent of people with depression are at the same time diagnosed with an anxiety disorder. Another huge study has found that, in 62 percent of all cases, it was actually a different mental disorder that set off a person's depression (and, let it be noted, there are few things more stressful than a mental illness).

Genes and Depression

There is a major genetic component to depression, too. Depression often runs in the family, and not merely as a consequence of depressive parenting. If one identical twin develops depression, the probability that the other twin—who shares 100 percent of his DNA, and nearly 100 percent of his family environment—will have a major depressive episode during his lifetime is about 45 percent. On the other hand, if a fraternal twin develops depression, the probability that the other (non-identical) twin—who shares only 50 percent of his DNA, but the same 100 percent of his family environment—will have a major depressive episode during his lifetime is just over 20 percent. Although these percentages vary somewhat across different twin studies taken from different populations, the overall pattern remains the same: identical twins have a higher concordance rate for depression than non-identical twins, and non-identical twins have a higher concordance rate than the lifetime prevalence of the disorder in the population at large.

Genes do not cause depression, but confer vulnerability to depression in the face of a difficult life. Scientists have discovered one crucial gene, involved in the synthesis of a serotonin-transporting protein, that affects vulnerability to depression in a major way. The gene exists in two variants: a more-efficient, long variant, and a less-efficient, short variant. Because we have two copies of practically every gene, a person can have three possible combinations of these two versions: two long versions, two short versions, and one long and one short version. A groundbreaking longitudinal study, which followed over a thousand New Zealanders from birth to adulthood, examined how this particular gene, and the number of major life-stressors a person experienced after his twenty-first birthday, but before his twenty-sixth birthday, affected his chances of developing depression in his twenty-seventh year. It found that, in subjects with no history of depression before age twenty-one, all three genotypes had the same ten percent chance of developing depression, but only if they encountered zero major life-stressors. In subjects who did experience major life-stressors, however, the difference clearly emerged: every stressor increased the likelihood of developing depression by 2 percent in persons with two long versions of the gene, by 4 percent in those with a long and a short version, and by 8 percent in those with two short versions—so that, in the subjects who encountered four or more major life-stressors, their rates rose to 18 percent in the long-long genotype, to nearly 30 percent in the long-short genotype, and to over 40 percent in the short-short genotype. This appears to be the way all relevant genes shield or predispose a person to depression, and to mental illness in general: by making certain psychological reactions either more or less likely in response to external events.

The heritability of depression—that is, the contribution to developing it that can be attributed to genetics (to nature rather than nurture)—has been placed at around 38 percent.

Unrecognized Depression

It used to be much more common, when depression wasn't a widely known term, that people suffering from it would not recognize there was something seriously wrong with them. They implicitly regarded their negative thoughts and dismal feelings as a regular and unavoidable part of their lives, and it was by no means obvious to them that this behavior was pathological. The nonfiction writer Lee Stringer describes this, from a time he was suffering from depression: "I knew something was wrong with my life. I was keenly aware of happiness becoming an increasingly elusive thing. A thing which, more and more, I couldn't grasp for any substantial length of time. But I didn't see anything unique about this. I simply put it down as a symptom of the human condition."[1]

Other depressed individuals, usually those with intense depressions, do see that something is direly wrong with them, but can't understand what it is. For many such people, a mere diagnosis produces tremendous relief, informing them that their various inexplicable symptoms—their emotional emptiness, feelings of worthlessness, desires for suicide, and all kinds of physical pains—are not indications of some permanent neurological malfunction or fatal disease, but the well-known signs of a common psychological malady: depression. This collapses the many terrifying possibilities they had hypothesized (and endlessly worried about) into a single, concrete, and addressable reality. And for those whose depression is mainly hormonal (like many post-partum depressions), this diagnosis alone relieves most of their misery, and then rapidly transitions to a full recovery.

Today, with the rather colloquial spread of knowledge about depression and mental illness, the failure to recognize depression has become much rarer—although it still occurs very often in young children.

Complaining or Secretive Depression

Some depressed persons make great efforts to hide their misery from others, especially if they don't realize that their condition is pathological. Others, on the other hand, actively—and often

---

[1] The term "depression," of course, is only a man-made concept, so it's perfectly natural that a person will fail to identify it in himself as a pathological malady. It's interesting to observe, though, how the self-centered nature of the human mind, making a person occupied with only his current thoughts and problems, can occlude a wider perspective that something about the nature of those thoughts and problems is fundamentally wrong.

unprovoked—announce their own misery, and self-loathing, and wishes for death, especially to close friends and relatives.

Bipolar Depression

Depression also has the very odd tendency, in some people, to be replaced with its exact opposite: mania (a state of intense joy, confidence, and excitement). But this almost invariably reverts back to depression, and the two emotional states typically alternate from one to the other over a period of weeks, days, or even minutes. In these cases, it is then classified as a different disorder: Bipolar.

Additional Symptoms

A few other commonly observed symptoms of depressed persons are that they are frequently on the verge of tears, they are extremely sensitive to rejection, they are overly concerned with other people's opinion of them, they lose the ability to find humor funny or laugh at jokes, they often inflict physical injuries on themselves, they sometimes harbor great anger toward some people without substantial reasons, and they frequently have a diminished sex drive, impotence, or an inability to orgasm. We have already made note of the other symptoms of affected sleep, appetite, a marked decrease in pleasure from activities, and the passive or active desire for suicide in the list of critical symptoms in the DSM.

Chapter 3

Causes

"Let us make no bones about it," writes Andrew Solomon. "We do not really know what causes depression." The list of symptoms and observations made of depressed people is certainly formidable, and not without some good clues as to the psychological nature of the condition. That is to be expected, as people have been observing depression for over two thousand years. But when it comes to the internal mental processes that lie behind the outwardly observable symptoms, as well as the causes of the illness as a whole, the present state of our understanding is still highly general and obscure.

As psychotherapist Gary Greenberg points out in *Manufacturing Depression: The Secret History of a Modern Disease*, the dialogue as to what causes depression, at least in the United States, has been hijacked today by the psychiatrists—the people of the book (the book being the DSM)—primarily because of the recent (though not unmixed) success achieved by treating the malady with anti-depressants, which only they, as medical doctors, are able to prescribe. But while the DSM "hinges on the elimination of theory," on cataloging the varieties of mental illness "without any comment on where it comes from, what it means, or what ought to be done about it," it has in the process tacitly substituted its own one-dimensional theory: that depression is the result of chemical imbalances in the brain, a purely organic, biological disease just like diabetes or cancer.

The more sophisticated psychologists, however, adopt what's now called a biopsychosocial perspective—which contends that a person's biology, his mental processes, and the social and physical conditions under which he lives, all play their own part and interact with each other (in various complicated, multidirectional ways) to produce the mental disorder of depression. That much is undeniably true—and I have depicted this model in *Figure 1*.

(1) We certainly know that the external environment, both social and physical, can affect psychology. Traumatic events in a person's life—including adverse childhood experiences, rejection by a real or potential lover, the diagnosis of a serious illness, and the death of a loved one—as well as his own long-term behavior—like involvement in an abusive, dependent, or jealous relationship; living a lonely, isolated lifestyle; or getting addicted to drugs, gambling, or alcohol—can produce serious psychological changes in the person, which can both trigger and predispose him to getting depression.

(2) These psychological changes—including grief, hopelessness, worry, guilt, self-blame, repressed emotions, and reduced self-esteem—can then produce biological changes, like alterations of hormone and neurotransmitter levels, that can lead to the physical symptoms of depression (including disturbed sleep, disturbed appetite, and lethargy). They can also produce *other* psychological changes—like anhedonia (the inability to experience pleasure), cognitive distortions, and suicidal impulses—that are the psychological symptoms of depression. And they can produce many behavioral changes, including a host of self-defeating tendencies, which alter the way the person interacts with his surroundings, and can lead to further traumatic events, as well as long-term patterns of self-destruction.

(3) In the meantime, the person's biology can play its own critical role. In some rare cases, a purely biological disorder—including Parkinson's disease, hypothyroidism, hypoglycemia, diabetes, and renal failure—can directly induce the psychology of depression. Genetic factors can predispose a person to depression. And changes in neurotransmitter levels, hormone levels, and brain

structure—themselves initially caused by psychology—will themselves go on to affect psychology, and in a way that can set off depression.

But while all of this is, once again, perfectly true, it's also extremely low-resolution. There now exist thousands of academic papers on the biology of depression (by far the most studied aspect of the disorder)—on the hormone levels, the neurotransmitter levels, the brain structure, and the regions of brain activation found in depressed persons—but nobody really knows how this biology affects psychology; and they have only the vaguest idea of how psychology affects biology. There is a fair amount of "Life Events" research into depression—into the types of events that trigger or predispose a person to the disorder—but the cognitive mechanisms by which these events operate, and the psychological impressions they leave on a person's mind, are still only subjects of tentative inference. As usual, psychology is the weakest link. And the nuanced interactions between the different parts of a person's mental life—in other words, the very meat of depression—are rarely even acknowledged, let alone understood. *That* is what I intend to elucidate in this book.

– The Biopsychosocial Model –

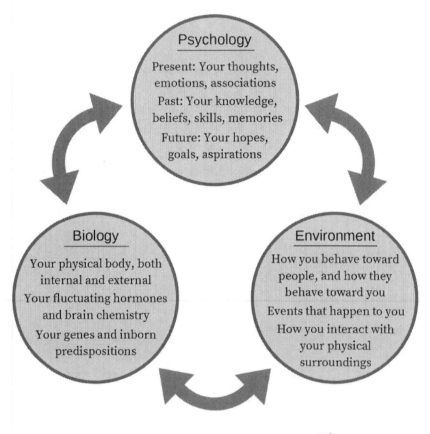

Psychology
Present: Your thoughts, emotions, associations
Past: Your knowledge, beliefs, skills, memories
Future: Your hopes, goals, aspirations

Biology
Your physical body, both internal and external
Your fluctuating hormones and brain chemistry
Your genes and inborn predispositions

Environment
How you behave toward people, and how they behave toward you
Events that happen to you
How you interact with your physical surroundings

Figure 1

Chapter 4

Treatments

Although "we have made but small advances in our understanding of depression," writes Andrew Solomon, "we have [nevertheless] made enormous advances in our treatment of depression."

Indeed, depression today is highly treatable, and by a wide variety of methods. All of these methods can and do lead to genuine improvement in a large number of depressed people, but they all also leave lots to be desired.

Medication

Depression is now treated primarily with drugs: antidepressants, as well as drugs that address other symptoms (such as sleeplessness, anxiety, and concentration). There are, as of this writing, over sixty different kinds of antidepressants—which says a lot about their efficacy. They aren't very predictable drugs. All of them work somewhat better than a placebo, but not by much. Any given depressed person, on any given antidepressant, has only a marginally better chance of improving than on a regular sugar pill—a significant reduction of symptoms in about 30 to 40 percent of cases, when it comes to the sugar pill.

But while no antidepressant is much more effective than any other, each is effective with a different segment of the population.

This means that, while no single drug has a very good chance of producing improvement, the entire arsenal of over sixty of them does. If one pharmaceutical fails to work, psychiatrists will—by trial and error—keep on prescribing their patient a different drug, until one of them finally has the desired effect. Usually, with enough time and trials, the doctor will eventually find a drug (or combination of drugs) that provides real relief for the patient's illness.

The biggest and most thorough study of antidepressant treatments, the STAR*D, found that about 67 percent of depressed patients who didn't quit taking their medication experienced a total remission of their symptoms after a maximum of four trials. This news, however, isn't all good. Half of the patients who experienced remission in the study relapsed after twelve months. Furthermore, the drugs often have awful side-effects—including nausea, weight gain, blurred vision, fatigue, vertigo, and erectile dysfunction—leading many patients, about 42 percent in the STAR*D study, to abandon their treatment. On top of all that, those who do benefit from the drugs become dependent on them, and their depression usually returns if they try to go off the pills, along with a mass of withdrawal symptoms. As a result, many people on antidepressants end up having to take them once a day, every day, for the rest of their lives.

Psychological Cures

While detailed first-hand (or even second-hand) accounts of something causing a person's depression are enigmatically rare in the literature, analogous accounts of something curing a person's depression are practically nonexistent. Still, several concrete types of event—whether a purely internal event, or an internal event caused by an external event—have been known to cure people's depression, and I will list these psychological cures here.

One psychological cure to depression is a corrective experience. Richard O'Connor gives the example of General Tecumseh Sherman, a prominent Union general in the American Civil War. Sherman was, to quote Richard O'Connor, a "textbook case" of a lifelong depressive, who contracted "a full-blown major depressive episode early in the Civil War." A standout graduate from the West Point military academy, he found himself in command of an army division at the start of the Battle of Shiloh, where his "life and character changed" profoundly, and which "cured his depression permanently."

The enemy launched a surprise attack in the morning hours, and succeeded in catching the Union forces off guard. Not having the time to even become anxious, Sherman instinctively leaped into action, and fought expertly and courageously for both days of the bloody battle, despite getting wounded twice and having three of his horses shot out from under him. Sherman was instrumental in forcing the enemy into retreat, became a war hero overnight, and decisively proved his ability to himself and to everyone around him.

This type of powerful experience, which—beyond any possible doubt—corrects some gross misperception, or resolves some burning uncertainty concerning oneself, the world, or other people (including doubts about one's self-worth) is one thing that can cure a depression. In Sherman's case, this type of experience—which proves a vital fact to oneself (and, as an added bonus, to other individuals)—also satisfied two of his basic, cognitive human needs: for self-esteem and the respect of his peers (which was, incidentally, the primary conflict of his depression).

Another psychological cure of depression can come from a purely internal, self-contained realization. The 19th century English philosopher John Stuart Mill, who's autobiography contains the best introspective account of depression I have found anywhere, thoroughly details how he attained such a cure. His depression centered around his conclusion that reforming society and government, which was his main "object in life," so that all people would in some distant future be "free and in a state of physical comfort," would also eliminate all pleasures from human existence—just like his own anhedonia—given that pleasure was only attainable through conquering "struggle and privation." It was cured, completely and permanently, due to an acute pleasure he unexpectedly experienced from reading some poetry, "which had no connection with struggle or imperfection," and which led him to realize that there still would be "perennial sources of happiness, [even] when all the greater evils of life . . . have been removed."

A third type of cure for depression, part psychological and part physical, can come from escaping some serious peril, or—on the positive end—obtaining some object one desperately needs or desires. The 20th century Soviet novelist, historian, and Nobel Prize winner Aleksandr Solzhenitsyn, for instance, was fully cured of his first and only major depressive episode by physically escaping his house in the Soviet Union, where "almost every night I fully expected to be arrested," and which was the central crisis of his depression, making all action and striving utterly pointless. Other people's depressions have been cured by obtaining a much-needed job, or starting a romantic relationship, or—in the case of one Cambodian farmer who lost his leg to a landmine—being gifted a cow. (In the Cambodian's case, his injury made farming the rice paddies an excruciating endeavor, and the cow let him make the career change from rice farmer to dairy farmer, a job he successfully managed despite missing a limb.)

Talk Therapy

Given that there exist psychological cures to depression, psychotherapy—whether tacitly or overtly—tries to obtain them in depressed patients.

Psychotherapy (or *talk* therapy) is the holistic, nonchemical alternative for treating depression. As with antidepressants, there are many different types of talk therapy—Psychoanalysis (which focuses on understanding the past origins of the patient's psychological problems), Interpersonal Therapy (which focuses on examining and improving the patient's relationships with other people), Cognitive Behavioral Therapy (which focuses on changing the patient's maladaptive thinking-patterns and beliefs), and various others—all of which, strangely enough, are about equally effective in treating depression. This equal effectiveness of all therapies has been labeled the "dodo bird effect:" something that apparently results from the success of a treatment depending, more than anything else, on the quality of the therapist and the relationship formed between him and the patient. The most important thing in a therapist, writes Andrew Solomon, is "intelligence and insight," while "the type of insight," the therapeutic techniques, and the theoretical structure used "are really secondary."

Not only are all therapies about as effective as one another, but therapy alone is about as effective as antidepressants alone, and both are just slightly more effective than a placebo.

Antidepressants plus Therapy

But while neither antidepressants or therapy are very effective as standalone treatments, the combination of antidepressants and therapy is. Around 80 percent of patients will experience significant improvement with therapy and medication combined.

The biggest benefit of medication, it seems, is making the patient motivated enough to attend therapy. And therapy, writes Andrew Solomon, "allows a person to make sense of the new self he has attained on medication."

Electroconvulsive Therapy

Interestingly enough, the combination of therapy and medication is about as effective as a third type of treatment: Electroconvulsive Therapy (ECT). Nowadays, this merely consists of a second-long shock to a single hemisphere of the patient's brain while he's placed in a ten-minute coma under an anesthetic. A full course of treatment consists of ten-to-twelve sessions spread out over six weeks. This is effective, at least in significantly reducing symptoms, over 75 percent of the time, and is typically used for individuals with severe depression (but it does include memory loss as an unpleasant side-effect).

Why Are Treatments So Ineffective?

The efficacy of depression treatments, of course, is highly under-whelming. Even when a treatment is successful, whether through therapy, medication, or both, the recovery it typically produces, states Richard O'Connor, is a "return to the same comfortable state of misery [the person] endured before [his] depression became un-bearable." A genuine state of wellbeing, O'Connor continues, "is the very last step of recovery," and a step most depressed patients will never reach.

There are, as we'll see, many legitimate reasons for this—for the existing treatments for depression being frequently unsuccessful, temporary, or partial. One major reason, however, is a poor under-standing of the psychology of depression, and what is really needed to cure it. Another is, to quote Andrew Solomon, the fact that de-pression is "a peculiar assortment of conditions" grouped under the same heading, with "a whole catalog" of different causes, and for each of which one type of treatment might be a lot more appropriate than others. Each type of talk therapy, for example, could be quite effective for a limited subset of those depressions, with their own particular causes and obstacles, but not for others.

A better understanding—both of the in-depth, psychological in-tricacies of depression and its range of possible subtypes and varia-tions—can therefore be used to improve treatment approaches as well. And that is what this book will provide: an improved under-standing of the nature and diversity of depression, rooted in personal insights obtained through introspective psychology.

Chapter 5

Deconstructing Depression

In seeking to understand depression, we should first form a clear picture of its psychological profile. We can do this best by starting from a solid foundation: not by trying to explain and incorporate all that we know of it, all at once; but by starting with what we know with the greatest certainty, and painting our picture of depression, layer by layer, from the bottom up. So, let us begin with what we undoubtedly know.

The Core of Depression

The chief facet that gives depression its character is undoubtedly the emotion of sadness; and without the emotion of sadness, there wouldn't be any question of depression.

Indeed, there is no better description of the essence of depression than a persisting and continually occurring sadness. The sadness recurs in pangs, or waves, and the severity of the condition is determined by how often they occur, how long they last, and how intense the actual feeling of sadness is. (Later, as the depression progresses, the peaks and troughs of the waves begin to gradually flatten out and remain at a constant, persistent level, becoming no longer pangs but a baseline numbness, less a feeling and more an "inability to feel," so that—in the words of Andrew Solomon—the "sadness as you had known it, the sadness that seemed to have led you here," transforms instead—to quote Richard O'Connor—into "a big heavy blanket that insulates you from the world yet hurts at the same time.") The general intensity of the sadness varies from person to person and case to case, and (from what we know about the way feelings affect behavior) it is precisely this intensity that is responsible for how debilitated the person becomes when he is struck with a depressive episode.[2]

The person will also experience a disproportionately huge drop (upon contracting the illness, as it were) in his ability to derive satisfaction, enjoyment, pleasure, from nearly all activities, even those that he used to enjoy: an anhedonia.[3] As a result, the person eventually loses interest in almost all prospective activities, and since the thought of practically every activity is now met with indifference and dread, it causes many people suffering from depression to eventually become confined to their own homes.[4] Often, however, at least at

---

[2] If the sadness is of a lower intensity, it will fully inhibit only the less motivated, frivolous, unessential activities of the person's daily life. He'll still retain the capacity to perform his more and most important activities, including his job and social obligations. But even then, the feeling of sadness and its displeasure will definitely remain, and make performing those duties a painful and stressful experience—in doing which the person may feel as though he's lifting a giant boulder. When, on the other hand, the sadness is of a much greater intensity (even in the same person, and with all other factors remaining equal), it can make the whole range of his activities totally impossible, and render him barely capable of performing the most basic biological functions.

[3] We can expect this kind of effect solely on the basis of a constantly lurking displeasure, which the person is condemned to feel as a result of his sadness. This makes even activities that were previously pure bliss for him an intermixture of pleasure and pain. But the effect is much greater than that. It's as if the inherent benefits of the activities themselves—the victories, the joys, the conquests—have become greatly devalued for the person. In effect, not only is an element of pain peppered into the pleasure of his activities, but the very pleasure that the activities used to provide is itself chopped down and depleted of intensity.

[4] The depressed person is, in fact, fully justified in losing interest in all prospective activities—given that he anticipates (and usually quite correctly)

the beginning of the illness, there will be one particular kind of activity or topic that is not met with the same characteristic indifference and despondency by the depressed person.[5]

In the progression of a depressive episode, if it isn't improved or alleviated, it will typically worsen, with the waves of the person's sadness growing more constant, closer together, and more intense.[6] Thoughts and compulsions to commit suicide will frequently occupy

---

that he will not derive any pleasure from them, and instead only have a painful and stressful time. He isn't always correct in this assumption; and we know it to be untrue for especially engrossing activities that leave the person with no opportunity to indulge his pathological thoughts: they take his mind off of his problems, and in the meantime provide some level of enjoyment. Still, the benefit of these activities will be retroactively devalued by the depressed person, and the enjoyment they provided won't last very long after the activity is over. So, even in these cases, the person ends up feeling that the effort it takes him to overcome his initial dejection and participate in an activity, even one that he knows will bring him some pleasure, does not warrant engaging in it: The juice, to this person, is not worth the squeeze.

[5] In some cases it is met, in great contrast, with eagerness or interest (most often at the initial phases of the illness); in other instances it is also met with disdain, but one that is quite peculiar and irregular—perhaps with guilt, or shame, or anxiety, or anger—as compared to the attitude taken toward all other subjects. This uncharacteristic attitude should be evident to the careful observer, and the actual topic varies from person to person. It is my strong suspicion that behind this abnormal topic usually lies the primary cause of a person's depression.

[6] We have to attribute this to new experiences in the depressed person's life that occur during the period of his illness, and which add on to those that initially caused it. After all, the depressed person quickly acquires more and bigger reasons to set off the bouts of his sadness (as well as his other negative emotions), in the variety of pains, fears, and disappointments inherent in the seemingly miserable, hopeless, and impotent life he now leads—and which his original depression is no doubt the cause of. (This is the classic downward spiral of depression.) We also can't overlook, however, a steady weakening of the constitution—an increased stress reactivity—that occurs in the depressed person, and which results from the constant strain of having to bear a huge amount of displeasure.

the person's mind, as his only foreseeable means of relieving this psychological anguish.[7]

The Emotion of Sadness

Having formed a clear picture of depression's key elements, we can set to unraveling its psychological causes. We will start by probing deeper into the emotion of sadness, which is undoubtedly at the core of this mental disorder.[8]

Sadness, like all the emotions, is an inborn affective response that gets automatically triggered whenever we experience pleasure or displeasure in a certain situational context.[9] For example: Anger is evoked whenever we recognize an external object—people and animals included—as being the cause of our displeasure. Sadness, on the other hand, arises due to the loss of something that was once a source of pleasure. This isn't limited to the loss of an object; and very often it occurs from the loss of a pleasurable idea, the loss of an expectation of pleasure, the loss of hope. There is no doubt that sadness, or at least some amount of sadness, is always evoked by the death of a loved one. It is also evoked by the loss of something a lot more trivial, like when a child is overcome with sadness and instantly

---

[7] There can also be other, peripheral motivations for suicide. And I will discuss these later on in the book.

[8] To clear up one point of potential confusion about sadness and anhedonia in the DSM: Although the DSM-5 requires that *either* (1) a sad or "empty" mood for most of the day nearly every day, *or* (2) a loss of interest or pleasure in all, or practically all, activities be present for a diagnosis of major depression, it later clarifies that that's not because anhedonia will sometimes be present in the absence of sadness, but because a depressed person will sometimes lose "the ability to describe [his] emotions (alexithymia)," become so numb that he no longer notices his emotions, or be unable to acknowledge that he is sad "for cultural or other reasons." "In almost all cases," however, "the person will be able to admit to the loss of interest or pleasure." (The DSM-5 Guidebook, page 111)

[9] To prevent confusion on the part of the reader, I wish to underline the meaning of the word "affect." Affect, *noun* – An internal feeling. Do not mistake it for the *verb* affect, meaning to have an influence on.

breaks into tears upon dropping his ice-cream cone.[10] In much the same way, we can observe how even a fully grown man is suddenly and easily brought to the verge of tears: when, in a lighthearted attempt to bring some small joy to a friend, partner, or child—while acting on the purest of intentions, and having nothing but warm, positive expectations—his kindly gesture is met, instead, by an offhand rejection or insult.[11]

We also know that a similar loss of a future prospect of pleasure, a loss of hope, also invariably produces sadness: like when a person receives confirmation that a childhood friend he looked forward to seeing won't be attending their high school reunion. And it is evident that many situations of loss actually contain a confluence of these factors: a loss that is simultaneously of something physical and something prospective. (The death of a loved one, for example, is rarely

---

[10] The saying: "Do not cry over spilled milk" serves in fact as a rational correction of an emotional response, because it is precisely a loss of this sort that instinctively triggers the emotion of sadness. Most of us, I am sure, have had occasion to experience this type of reaction and can commiserate with the person who, when reaching for a glass of fresh milk with nothing but an innocent desire to drink it—to enjoy its cold, refreshing texture, to quench his growing thirst—instead fumbles and accidentally knocks it over, spilling onto the floor the entirety of the cold liquid that once promised to provide him with such a simple, carefree enjoyment.

[11] This raw, unmitigated sadness response, which comes on with no warning or explanation, appears to be due precisely to that person being utterly unprepared for this type of rebuff. He is caught off guard, as it were, by something that so blatantly defies his expectation. Indeed, this effect will not occur with nearly the same fervor when the person recognizes and is prepared for the possibility of a negative outcome, too—although he'll likely still experience some amount of sadness.

(There's no doubt that expectation, and the role it plays in the unconscious mind, is a central part of human psychology. It is the upsetting of expectation, which in the above scenario leads to sadness, that also leads—in a different context—to the joy and laughter we derive from humor. And it is the fear caused by a sudden emergence of a great danger, without it being anticipated by anxiety, that frequently leads to the traumas—such as those incurred by soldiers during a war—that later result in Post-Traumatic Stress Disorder.)

only the loss of a person who was the source of many happy and warm moments in the past; it is also the loss of somebody who promised to bring many more happy moments in the future.)

We can assume that the magnitude of the loss, or rather the thing that was lost, strongly corresponds to the magnitude of the sadness it will evoke.

The causes we listed above are the psychological source of what we may call primary sadness: a first-hand emotional response to a manifest situation in one's present environment. But like all emotions, it can also be evoked in a second-hand manner, by unconscious association.[12] This kind of second-hand emotion is experienced when a person perceives something—something that he sees, hears, tastes, smells, feels, or even thinks—that reminds him, even if he doesn't consciously realize it, of the event in which that emotion was evoked in its original, primary manner.[13] The emotion of sadness is no exception to this rule.

It was Freud who first formulated this insight, and psychologists have been using it ever since: That the precipitating causes of depression are no different from those that cause regular sadness. They come in the form of a loss, exactly as we described above. Often it

---

[12] It is the fundamental functionality of our unconscious mind to automatically provoke a recollection of past events, along with their originally-felt affects, when we presently experience something which bears a similarity to them. Similarity is, of course, the core mechanism by which the unconscious mind forms associative links between memories and novel perceptions.

[13] His awareness of the underlying source of this emotion can vary from a profound and detailed reminiscence of the original event, to nothing but the re-experiencing of the emotion itself, unaccompanied by any signs of the memory it stems from—as well as all the possible gradations between the two.

is the loss of a romantic relationship, the loss of a close friend or family member, or the loss of some hope or aspiration.[14]

We must conclude, then, that there is nothing irregular about the actual sadness experienced by the depressed person. Its psychological causes, as well as its effects, are exactly the same as those of ordinary, non-pathologized sadness: which can be experienced by all healthy people, as well as animals.

In light of this, it's most correct to view the factor separating depression from regular sadness to be, not the nature of the sadness itself, but the fact of its obstinate persistence; which is also undeniably what makes this affliction so pathological. We will proceed with our investigation by examining the psychological processes by which a person gets over a loss, and the sadness associated with it, and attempt to determine what factors are present (or absent) in the depressed person that could inhibit this from occurring.

Reevaluation

We know from Freud that a strong emotion instigated by primary means will be preserved alongside the memory of its provoking event and re-experienced with roughly all its original fervor whenever that event is recalled. However, this will only occur if the person was (and still is) unable to act on that emotion or resolve it in some other way.[15] In such cases, the act of recalling the event will, as a rule,

---

[14] There are many cases in which a person attributes the cause of his depression to a different kind of source. But upon probing the issue with sufficient depth, we consistently find such an assessment to be mistaken, and that the event triggering the depression really did involve some type of loss, but one that the person wasn't aware of. Occasionally, this realization alone can be the cure for depression. And in cases where no cause of the depression can be found, we have good reason to believe that at their core, too, lies a loss of this nature, only one that remains unidentified.

[15] A great example of this is anger. It is the person who holds a grudge, because he was unable to get revenge on somebody that once harmed him, who re-experiences his original anger when he remembers that villainous person or the injury that was dealt to him. Every time he recalls this, he

be performed less and less vividly over time, until it becomes little but an unconscious association, with only the emotion itself being felt and the original causes becoming vague and forgotten. The magnitude of the emotion will typically diminish in strength, but never subside fully, as the unconscious memory of it becomes increasingly obscure.

There are two ways a person can free himself from this kind of emotional stigmata. The first is performing the built-in action that each emotion innately urges him to commit. Anger urges a person to exact revenge on whatever that anger is directed at. Anxiety urges a person to prepare himself for, or to otherwise avoid, whatever situation provokes it. Excitement urges a person to seek out in reality the object or activity that excites him. And as for the emotion of special importance to us in this book: sadness, produced by loss, urges a person to regain or replace what is lost. If the person is successful in carrying out these actions, the provoking emotion will be satisfied and the memory of the event that caused it will be purged of its emotional charge.

The second way this can happen is through a conscious reevaluation of the event itself, which is the result of a special reframing of

---

wants revenge once more. But if he at some point succeeds in getting his revenge, the anger will subside, and he will no longer experience any anger toward that person, or in response to the thoughts and memories which had—before his revenge—never failed to rouse that resentment. And had he avenged himself right as the original anger was incurred, he wouldn't have had to deal with any persisting feelings of anger in the first place. It is important, however, that the revenge be of an adequate retribution for the incurred injury; otherwise, some feelings of anger will still remain.

A similar effect of letting go of a grudge and purging residual anger is often produced when the person confesses his anger, talks it out, and comes to terms with it. At those times, the person forgives the villain and comes out no longer blaming the man for his injury. Then too, thoughts of that person or the injury will cease to be laden with anger; although it isn't uncommon, in those cases, for there to be an occasional relapse, with some anger once again being felt upon recalling the topic (though only sporadically, and without resurrecting the grudge).

that occurrence in the person's mind, a process that strongly appeals to us for its therapeutic value. It's only natural to assume that by understanding it we can gain the ability to cure depression—and many other psychological troubles besides. That's what we will examine next.

One common situation where this type of reframing occurs is in the person flooded with sadness after the death of a parent. There isn't much this person can do, after all, to fulfill the instinctual imperative brought onto him by the sadness: to replace what he lost. What substitute can there really be for a mother or a father? With this first means of getting over his sadness closed off to him, the person has only the second option left, lest the loss of his parent remain a psychological stigma that he must live with for the rest of his life. Yet we can be sure, at least for the majority of cases, that he will indeed get over it and eventually come to accept the fact of his parent's death with serenity. And this truly is the result we see in most healthy people who have experienced the death of a parent.

We can obtain lots of insight into what reevaluating an emotional event really entails, if we examine in detail the mental processes of the person coping with a parent's death, from the time of his loss to the time that he comes to peace with it. What occurs in a person during this time is a period of profound bereavement very similar in its symptoms to clinical depression. Indeed, this period of grief can last several years, and the mourner will likewise experience a general and pervasive sadness, and the same factor that causes it (the death of a parent) will often cause major depression in other people. However, this period of grief, which we consider a perfectly normal part of human existence, lacks some of the key features of pathological depression—which I will discuss later. And while we can expect grief to improve over time and then naturally come to an end, we frequently expect depression to take a more sinister course—and therefore require some medical intervention.

Our preliminary impression, then, is that some added factor (or factors) are present in depression, but absent in regular grieving, which work to prevent or invalidate the cognitive reappraisal that normally heals the latter but not the former. We will examine this later as well.

Framing and the Emotional Response

But before we attempt to make sense of reevaluation, or the thought processes that facilitate it in the grieving person, we should first answer a different question: Why is an emotion, at one time caused by a highly emotional event, from then on automatically reproduced, and with almost all its original intensity, whenever that event is recalled?

The popular theory is that the emotion becomes unconsciously associated, in memory, to the event in which it was initially experienced. But this doesn't explain why the emotion (or mix of emotions) a memory evokes can be permanently removed or even replaced with different emotions by means of some action, a new set of circumstances, or cognitive reappraisal. This simply doesn't accord with the normal functions of associative memory. In no other case can a formed association be retroactively erased or transformed, by any means.

Instead, we can understand this phenomenon when we look at it from the following perspective. First, we need not assume there is any fundamental difference between the way an emotion is evoked primarily, in response to an original event, and how it's evoked secondarily, in response to the event's memory. Then, we need only grant that, as long as the memory of that event remains unchanged and undergoes no reinterpretation or shift in perspective, the person will effectively re-live the event (reproducing it over and over again in its original form) every time he recalls it.[16] Since the memory

---

[16] And when this act of remembering the event becomes less and less vivid with time, leaving behind mostly unconscious (though still emotion-filled) associations, we may say that the person no longer needs to re-live the event, because he already knows what will happen (or rather, what has happened) and reacts accordingly.

essentially provides the same input as the original event and will continue to do so each time it's recalled, it will each time evoke the same emotion—or mix of emotions—anew.

This perspective appears to be the correct one. We know that an emotion is evoked by instinct, automatically, when a person experiences pleasure or displeasure in a certain context; but it is the person's own mental interpretation of the event that creates this context. We likewise know that the way a person frames or evaluates an event is responsible for the emotion that situation elicits, or whether it elicits any emotion at all.[17] It is undeniable that this kind of interpretation, once made, becomes unconsciously tied to the actual facts

---

[17] As Seymour Epstein noted in his incredible book *Constructive Thinking: The Key to Emotional Intelligence*, different people can interpret the same event in different ways and feel, as a result, a different emotion. In a psychology class he taught at the University of Massachusetts, he performed an exercise in which one student had to recall a situation from his past when he reacted with a strong emotion, and then the rest of the class responded with how they would react if they were put in the same situation.

He gives the example of one student, Robert, who recalled the following incident: His mother and father were getting a divorce, and both were trying to win Robert over to their side, to convince him that everything was the other parent's fault, and constantly accusing him "of siding with the other parent." One day, when Robert came home to pick up some warm winter clothes, he found only his mother at home. She had locked all the doors, refused to let him inside, and yelled at him through the window "that he deserved such treatment because he sided with his father."

Robert's strongest emotion, he said, was anger, "and his thoughts preceding the emotion were that his mother had no right to treat him that way, that she was being unfair because he had not sided with his father," and whatever the case might have been, that simply was "no way for a mother to treat her son." He was fully convinced that everyone else, if exposed to the same situation, would experience anger as well.

A show of hands from the class, however, demonstrated otherwise. Out of the fifteen students in the class, ten did say they would react with anger, but two said they'd react with sadness, "one with fear, one with sympathy, and one with cool detachment and perhaps even amusement." This wide diversity of responses "absolutely amazed" Robert. "The angry reaction was so natural to him that he could not [even] imagine" a different response.

of the event and affects the way that a person remembers it: A person will remember an emotional event not in isolation, but in the context of how it personally affected and/or continues to affect him or her.

Thus, we have the true nature of the psychological mark an emotional event leaves on a person: It is really, not the emotion itself, but his interpretation of the event that the person subconsciously retains. And it is this interpretation, and not the emotion, that will later unconsciously transpose itself onto situations similar to that original event.

This is actually a very interesting and important psychological phenomenon, because every emotional event that comes to hold significance for a person (often being significant due to the very fact that it was highly emotional) serves a kind of nucleating role in

---

A female student who said her strongest emotion was sadness said that her "automatic thoughts preceding the emotion" were that she would feel "pretty worthless" if her own mother began treating her this way. She would think that she "deserved" such treatment because of something she did, such as "not being a loving enough daughter."

The one student who reported she would feel fear said that "her thoughts preceding the emotion" were that her mother's behavior was that of a crazy person, and that the mother might be planning to harm her in other ways, and could "even attack her physically." Her first impulse would be "to get out of there" and decide what to do with the winter clothes at a later time.

The woman who said she would mainly feel sympathy described her thoughts before the emotion as: "someone would have to be very upset to behave so unreasonably." Her first impulse would be to give her mother time to calm down, and then sympathetically listen to what was bothering her. She would then do what she could to provide "emotional support," and tell her mother "how much she loved her."

The male student who said his reaction would be a "cool detachment" and perhaps even amusement reported that he would find it "somewhat funny" that a grown adult could behave so irrationally, and "in a way that [was bad] for her health and would estrange herself from her own son." (*Constructive Thinking*, pp 27-28)

subconsciously imposing its interpretation on all similar events, not only in the future, but in the past as well.[18]

---

[18] When a person discovers that he has been cheated by a friend (let's say the friend stole something valuable from him), previously unemotional or even fond memories of interacting with that friend will now evoke anger, since he suddenly interprets them as preludes to the scam perpetrated on him, and sees his friend's past actions in the context of him harboring those very malevolent intentions that resulted in the betrayal. (This is, in itself, a reevaluation.)

Furthermore, once this initial evaluation is made, similar events in the future will *also* be subject to having that same interpretation unconsciously transposed upon them. For example: When this same person experiences a similar misfortune to the one his traitorous friend caused him, or merely suspects that he will (let's say he suddenly can't find his wallet), we can predict that he will react with anger and mistrust toward his *other* friends, suspecting them of being the cause of his new troubles—and doing so subconsciously and irrationally, in situations that in no way warrant this kind of suspicion, and where any unbiased person could only be expected to think of his friends as entirely innocent.

We know that the more meaningful or emotionally powerful the precipitating event, the greater will be its effect in transposing its interpretation onto similar situations and related memories. What makes this psychological phenomenon such a nuisance, and truly a huge factor in so many pathologies, is that the initial interpretation of the emotional event is usually *itself* unconscious and automatic—even without any past experiences bearing upon it. It can, of course, undergo conscious reevaluation and be logically corrected once this has occurred. But the person usually doesn't give it much thought or logical analysis, since he assumes it's already in the past and over with—and very often he is glad that it is. And by a grand peculiarity of human nature, people are naturally unaware of the mechanics of their unconscious psyche, having no idea of the extent to which such an event will influence their future emotions, thoughts, and experiences.

Unless it is made explicit to them, nearly all people will be completely oblivious to the fact that past experiences that aroused a great deal of emotion continue to play, and have continued to play since their inception, a major role in the way they react to and interpret the world. During therapy, people are taken by the greatest surprise when they realize an event they attributed no significance to has been tacitly influencing and directing their lives—their beliefs, their inhibitions, their insecurities, and so forth. But when they do realize this, they acquire a truly powerful amount of in-

This new perspective on the relation of emotion and memory also gives us a key insight into the cognitive reevaluation of a past event. It is essentially a conscious, corrective reappraisal of the way the event is framed in the person's mind, which was truly the decisive cause of its original emotionality in the first place. Once achieved, a reevaluation will essentially cause the person to remember that event in a different context.

The process of reevaluation can therefore transform one emotional response into another, produce an emotional response where there was none before, and convert a previously emotional situation or topic into a totally neutral or benign one. With that, let us return to our primary goal and examine in detail, as we intended, the process of reevaluation as it occurs in that strange period of mourning after the death of a parent.

---

sight; and in consciously understanding and logically reevaluating that crucial event (which they are now free to do), the insecurities, the fears, and all the other psychological products it spawned are shed almost instantly.

Chapter 6

Grief Following a Parent's Death

It was Freud, again, who first drew this parallel: that the psychological state of grief after the death of a loved one—especially a parent or spouse—is extremely similar to pathological depression. This was the meaning behind the title of his landmark essay: *Mourning and Melancholia*. The former, he wrote, would also appear highly bizarre and pathological to us, were it not such a commonplace, natural part of our lives.

There's one qualification I'd like to add here: In writing his seminal essay, Freud had in mind the sort of parental death and mourning experienced by a largely independent adult (perhaps like the death of his own father when Freud was forty, and after which he underwent a lengthy period of grief). Such a person may certainly love his mother or father, may highly appreciate all the care he or she took while raising him, may even maintain an intimate friendship with that parent right to the point of his or her death; but because the parent isn't an overly important part of that person's present life, his loss is a chiefly emotional, psychological one. In other cases, especially when it comes to children and adolescents, the loss of a parent can also mean the loss of a caregiver, the loss of a breadwinner, the loss of a safety net, and the loss of a best friend—in other words, it can mean a massive *physical* loss, in addition to an emotional, psychological one. The process of mourning, in that case, assumes an important additional dimension—or rather it amplifies one that is always present. It calls on the person to restructure his life, to adapt to these new, highly changed circumstances, on top of coming to peace with his parent's death. Freud overlooked this *practical* dimension of loss, along with any significance it might have for depression, much as he overlooked—in the same essay—that his depressed patients' frequently expressed fears of falling into poverty had any significance besides an unconscious regression to the "anal eroticism" of their toddlerhood. But while these practical repercussions of a loss certainly can, and do, play a large role in many people's depressions (and I will discuss these later), let's follow Freud's lead for now, and examine the kind of death Freud had in mind: that of an independent adult's mother or father, where the purely emotional, psychological component of grief is undiluted by coping with any extraneous, physical catastrophe.

The Psychology of Grief

Freud astutely observed that a person, following the death of a parent (a person in whom this event did not induce the clinical picture of depression), will have his mind predominantly occupied with thoughts and memories of that parent, which bring with them a considerable amount of sadness. It is with this activity of reminiscing that the period of bereavement is concerned, and the person becomes generally withdrawn and uninterested in the rest of the world in all of its aspects unrelated to the deceased loved one.

But this poses a curious theoretical dilemma for us. These odd reminiscences, after all, most clearly evoke a great deal of sadness in the person. And by the fundamental principles of the human unconscious, it is precisely the memories that evoke an unpleasant emotion that are compulsively resisted and avoided—this is, indeed, what happens to memories that provoke anxiety, shame, guilt, disgust, and (in many alternate cases) sadness—rather than instinctively sought after and indulged, as is the case in this scenario. Here, on the contrary, the unconscious mind appears to be treating these saddening thoughts and memories exactly as though they were pleasurable. Why?

Well, when we examine these reminiscences closer, we find that they really *are* pleasurable. And what brings these memories to mind in the first place is the aspect of warmth and happiness that they carry within them. (Indeed, it is widely acknowledged that the quality of such mournful reminiscences is frequently bittersweet, and not merely sad.) It is, of course, only now, after the loss of the loved one, that the memories of that person begin to evoke sadness. Earlier, those memories had been exclusively positive; only after his death do they acquire their new morose tint—since they are suddenly viewed under the light of *"that person who gave me such warm moments is now gone, and we will never be able to have such moments again,"* which as a result evokes sadness. This change in the emotionality of past events is clearly the outcome of a reevaluation.

We can discern another type of reevaluation here too. It's that even those memories of the deceased person that had earlier been entirely neutral—and regarded as irrelevant—now begin to evoke a pleasant fondness and warmth as well. It's as if the person whose sadness begs him to regain what was lost, attempts to regain his lost parent in the memories that he has of her. This is, in effect, a sort of tribute to the deceased: a revival of and reverence for her memory, which also serves as a reclamation of part of what was lost through her death. (In that roundabout way, the emotion of sadness—at least partially—accomplishes its intended, impossible goal: If it cannot replace what was lost *physically*, it will settle for doing so *psychologically*.)

Healthy Grief

In this way, the grieving person goes through a collection of memories of his parent and, at the end of this period of bereavement, emerges out of his grief and into a state of serene acceptance, and is then able to wholeheartedly resume his normal life. What occurs here is another reevaluation, but this time a conscious and rational one. And that this sort of reevaluation really did occur is apparent in the person's changed attitude, after the recovery, toward the loss, his memories, and death in general.

This person no longer views the death of his parent as a grave loss of somebody who was such a major part of his life, but—if we are to summarize the general view most people adopt—he grows to see his parent's existence as a persisting influence that benefited, affected, and shaped the course of his life, and which, as fate and nature has it, came to the natural end that all living things must at some point meet. It now looks like this reinterpretation is not just a way people cope with and overcome death, but a rich process of personal and intellectual development, which extends far past this single occurrence as a gained understanding of many other areas of life. The person comes out of this experience with a sort of wisdom; and indeed, we cannot deny the title of wisdom to the serene understanding and acceptance of death—not just his parent's, but death in general—that this person attained.

We can now recognize what role the person's remembrances play in leading him to this reassessment. It is during these recollections that the intellectual work of the reevaluation occurs. When we examine this process more closely, we find that the reminiscences don't merely consist of an uninvolved revisiting of a memory. On the contrary, they are of a thoroughly pensive, ruminating nature. The person evaluates and analyzes the memories to the fullest extent he can; and it is piece by piece, from each memory or cluster of memories, that he draws his conclusion that they aren't a relic of the beloved person he lost, but the various ways this person contributed to his life—and that the person may now be gone, but the happiness she brought, the memories she left, and the effect she had on his life isn't. When the mourner essentially exhausts his supply of memories and comes to terms with all or the most significant of them, only then does this new perspective extend to the actual death itself (along with all of its implications), which thereby allows him to overcome it.[19] (We can suppose that until this process is completed, the period of bereavement will continue; and that its duration depends on the time that it takes to carry it out to completion.)

A Wrench in the Griefwork

Let's now return to the subject of depression. We had concluded that the key element in depression was one that inhibited the curative function of reevaluation. Having examined this process of cognitive reassessment in detail, we should now have a much better idea of what these factors can be. Anything that inhibits the reminiscences, their rational deliberation, or the conclusions formed as a result suffices to meet that criterion. Certainly, influences that act as a drain on cognition or memory—which includes heavy drinking, substance abuse, psychosis, and perhaps even amnesia—will have this effect. In cases where such factors are present following a large loss, for example, if a person turns to drugs or alcohol to deal with the death of a parent, the sadness he experiences won't have a chance to be resolved, and we can regard this person as being, in all respects, in a state of depression—at least until he returns to sobriety, and becomes clearheaded enough to undertake the mental work of bereavement.

It is, however, clear that such are rather unusual cases of depression and make up a decided, though not insignificant, minority of all those that occur. (Drug or alcohol abuse is present in roughly 18 percent of depressed persons, and psychosis is present in roughly 14

[19] In his bestselling book, *12 Rules for Life,* the Canadian psychologist Jordan Peterson gives a compelling reason why this occurs. To consciously process a highly emotional event, like a love one's death, he says, "is often more about forgetting than about remembering." It is a process of sorting out the important, meaningful memories from the unimportant, inconsequential ones, until "the moral of the story"—"the central narrative" of the event—can be established. To do so, however, a person must first call up all of his relevant memories, and go through them one by one, needing—like a judge at a trial—to have all the evidence presented to him before he arrives at his final verdict. (See *12 Rules for Life*, page 247.)

percent—although, whenever these factors are present, treatment of the depression gets much more complicated, and its prognosis becomes much bleaker.) We must therefore search for another inhibiting factor that can have this effect, one that is present in the majority and the most typical cases of this disorder. And surely enough, precisely this type of factor is blatantly present, and just as blatantly observable, in the vast majority of people with major depression.

We can recognize this factor in an extremely peculiar behavior—a key symptom—that is so often present in clinical depression, but largely absent in normal grief after the loss of a parent, and in most other manifestations of regular sadness. This is the adamant self-denigration and reproachfulness that seems, to the outside observer, so striking and unjustifiable a characteristic of the depressed person. These people claim whole-heartedly that they are worthless, lowly, despicable; they speak of some vague, unspecified wrongdoings that they committed and repeatedly commit; they chide themselves for being a burden on their friends, partners, and relatives, who they decree should not even bother with someone as worthless as they are.[20]

Of course, to the observer this attitude appears entirely absurd and irrational, as so harsh a prognosis is hard to make of even the most detestable people. And on the contrary, it is too often easy to see in depressed persons the great aspects of beauty, intelligence, creativity, and potential. From a psychological standpoint, this behavior is even more enigmatic. For even in the most wicked people, of whom this kind of criticism may be considered appropriate, we find an exact opposite tendency toward self-esteem (rather than self-

---

[20] The depressed person's conviction about his own worthlessness is, as many of us have butted up against when dealing with a depressed friend or relative, entirely impervious to any logic, reason, or attempts to convince him otherwise. This is one thing he is fully certain of, and he can't be swayed from it by any direct method. Of course, this kind of blatant and stubborn irrationality is a rather common occurrence whenever we deal with anything in which emotions play a large part.

denigration), self-approval (rather than reproach), and an overvaluing of one's own person (rather than regarding oneself as worthless).

Indeed, this attitude in the depressed person runs completely contrary to the self-esteem seeking behavior that is such an instinctual part (at least in our more civilized societies) of normal human activity. And we know there is only one thing in the whole of the human psyche that can have this effect: It is the distinctive emotion of shame. But we also know of another inherent function of the emotion of shame: It urges the individual to avoid or abridge his thoughts and memories, specifically the thoughts and memories he is ashamed of. And this is, of course, exactly the kind of inhibiting factor we assumed was responsible, in persons suffering from depression, for preventing the mental work needed to consciously reevaluate a major loss.

Chapter 7

The Psychology of Shame: The Reproach Emotion

We seem to have reached the turning point of our investigation. Let us, then, examine in detail the emotion of shame, and see what insights it grants us into that vast majority of depressions that exhibit this symptom.[21]

I need to first make entirely clear what I mean by the emotion of shame. First off, the word "shame" is not the best fit to describe this emotion, although it is the nearest commonly used term that refers to it. Today, people confuse the words shame, guilt, and embarrassment, and often use the three interchangeably. But while the latter two terms are closely related to the emotion of shame, they are in fact markedly different, and refer to different emotional phenomena. In this book, the term I'll adopt to refer to it is "the reproach emotion," which I think is the most fitting.

I decided to name it "reproach emotion" because it's precisely reproach that evokes it. The emotion is triggered when a person remembers some prior misdeed of his, a past action he disapproves of or wishes he didn't commit. The physical feeling that comes with it

---

[21] Aaron Beck, in a survey of over seven hundred depressed patients, found that this kind of shame and "negative feelings toward [one]self" were present in 64 percent of patients with mild depression, in 81 percent of those with moderate depression, and in 86 percent of those with severe depression. (*Depression, Causes and Treatment*, page 17-19)

is an uncomfortable, heavy sensation around the pit of the stomach or solar plexus; it may feel like a drilling into, or an eating away, or a shaving away at that region of the body; some will describe it as a sudden blow to that area. It often causes the person to cringe or shudder (or at least want to) as a sort of physical effort to shake off, or knock away, the memory that evoked it.[22]

It is very common that a person experiencing this emotion will utter, whether in his mind or aloud, actual verbal reproaches in the form of single-phrase chants that condemn himself or his action. These phrases or chants serve the same purpose as does the wincing, cringing, or shuddering and are often expressed in conjunction with those gestures. Quintessential ones are: "God, that sucked," "I fuck-ing hate myself," "I'm a goddamn idiot," "Never again," "Thank God that's over," "Ugh." Usually, a person will have just one or two of these phrases he automatically recites to himself every time he recalls a reproachful event.[23]

---

[22] To return to the topic of guilt and embarrassment: Guilt, upon careful analysis, is not a separate emotion in itself, but a blend of the emotions of shame and anxiety. Embarrassment, on the other hand, is a completely separate instinctual reaction, one that can only be felt about something happening in the present (although recalling an embarrassing event can certainly, in retrospect, evoke shame, and being confronted about a prior reproachful action can certainly evoke embarrassment). There can't remain any doubt about the distinction between shame and embarrassment when we look at their physiological effects: The physical expression of embar-rassment induces a person to blush, to cover his face, to avoid people's gaze, whereas reproach does nothing of the sort, and (as we mentioned earlier) has totally different physical effects. Were we to name it after these, we may fittingly call it the "cringe" emotion.

[23] We may also observe that these phrases or chants are of the same nature as the self-hating reproaches expressed by the depressed person—with the exceptions that in the depressed person they are primarily directed at him-self (as opposed to his actions), they seem to be greatly elaborated upon, and they are held as static judgments of his own character, instead of ex-isting only in the brief moments that a shameful event is recalled.

The subject of the reproach emotion is always a person's own behavior, a behavior whose consequences carry with it some feeling of
displeasure. For the reproach emotion to be evoked, the person must
make the following evaluation of his already committed behavior: he
must view it as having been an incorrect or loathsome course of action, and perhaps just as importantly (indeed the reproach emotion
doesn't seem to occur without this) he must recognize a better alternative action that he could've taken at the time but didn't. Because
of this, unlike other emotions that are an instant response to a present event, the reproach emotion is usually experienced for the first
time in retrospect—often hours after the event, or the next day, depending on the time it takes for the person to draw the needed evaluation.[24] In fact, we can justly consider this a reevaluation of that past
event, since when that action was actually committed the person may
have had no emotional reaction to it whatsoever, or it might have
elicited a totally different emotion.

Common scenarios in which a person experiences the reproach
emotion are when he looks back at his behavior at a time of impaired
judgment (a time when he wasn't in his right mind). Often, it's his
perverse behavior during the heated moments of a sexual act (like
engaging in sultry or dirty talk, or taking certain sexual liberties with
the other person); or his belligerent behavior while he was intoxi-
cated (such as insulting somebody, or overzealously expressing his
fondness for them); or his short-sighted behavior during a state of
panic or nervousness (like running out on a restaurant bill when he
sees he's forgotten his wallet, or reactively lying to a person who

---

[24] It is, however, possible to experience the reproach emotion in time with
an event, as soon as the reproachful action is taken. An adolescent boy on
a date with a girl will have plenty occasions, right in the immediate moment,
to experience the painful reproach emotion (along with a suppressed desire
to wince, and a chiding phrase he may chant at himself—mentally, of
course, never aloud), right after he utters some unsuccessful joke, or when
the girl responds negatively to something he says. His evaluation that what
he said was a mistake, and that it would've been better had he not said it,
occurs instantly.

posed him an unexpected request or question); or even his self-pros-trating behavior over the course of some physical illness (such as vomiting, defecating, or lying down in a public place). In any case, it must be a behavior of which he's retroactively ashamed, and that he would not have committed if he had his wits about him, the way he does now when reflecting upon it.[25] But it's not unusual, even for the actions a person commits in his regular state of mind, to evoke the reproach emotion when he later apprehends them as foolish or flawed, and clearly sees the right course of action he should've taken.[26]

---

[25] It should be noted that most of the time during such periods of impaired judgment, the person feels no regret for his actions whatsoever. He only feels it later, after he regains his regular frame of mind. Interestingly, the individual's conscious knowledge that he wasn't in his right mind back then is outside the scope of the reproach emotion, and has essentially no bearing on it. He subconsciously sees his shameful behavior as the product of his own person, independent of the state of mind he was in.

[26] Good examples of this are:

1.) A student, after taking a math exam, realizes that he solved one of the problems incorrectly—then the proper solution dawns on him, and he sees that he knew how to get the correct answer all along, but failed to make that connection during the test. He imagines how easy it would've been to have gotten that right answer, and feels the reproach emotion.

2.) An experienced athlete makes a tactical error in a competitive sports match, and loses the game as a result. He realizes now what the correct play at the time should've been and that it was the clear choice in that situation. He imagines having made that play and winning the game instead, and feels the reproach emotion. (Interestingly, if the exact same scenario transpired, but the game was won despite it, the re-proach emotion would—for most people—never be evoked.)

3.) A teenage boy asks a girl out on a date, but is rejected because she already made plans with another boy. He later finds out that this other boy had asked her out only a day earlier: something that he himself was too nervous to do. He imagines asking the girl out a mere one day sooner, and feels the reproach emotion.

Consequences of Self-Reproach

The reproach emotion, like all emotions, has a built-in behavioral imperative: to aim at a redo. It urges the person to try placing himself in a nearly identical or analogous situation, and this time choose the correct course of action.[27] In this way, he seeks to amend his past folly, to right his past wrong. That motivation, however, is typically very short-lived. Most frequently, the reproachful event and the person's intention to amend it will only be held in his mind for a short time, before the opportunity for the redo is lost from sight and he is obliged to condemn it as unfeasible.[28] From that point, after the motivation to recreate the situation and correct his misdeed fades, the reproach emotion will only serve the auxiliary function of avoidance—as all unpleasant emotions and affects have the potential for doing. Specifically, it's the memory of the reproachful event that the person will adamantly avoid.

Once the initial evaluation linking an event with the emotion of reproach is made, the person will continue to experience that emotion alongside his memory of the event (until, of course, he reinterprets it or succeeds in amending his actions by behaving properly in an analogous scenario), and for only as long as the event is being recalled—remembering the painful event being, for him, the equivalent of reliving it. The psychological consequence is that the person

---

[27] Of course, what the person *actually* wants is to change the past: To have never committed the shameful action in the first place, and have instead done what he now sees as right. But since this is for obvious reasons impossible, he will seek in reality its nearest substitute, which is this type of corrective reenactment.

[28] The person frequently will, however, seek a transient satisfaction of this urge through the medium of his imagination. He will reproduce in his fantasies a scene similar to the original scenario where he committed his reproachful misdeed, and this time he will imagine acting as he wishes he acted then, and proceed to play that fictional situation out in his mind. (It is, of course, a common occurrence in human cognition for people to turn to fantasy and their imaginations as an illusory substitute for living out their unattained wishes and desires.)

needs only to avoid its memory to avoid the negative emotion. Whenever the memory of that event comes to mind, he will deliberately cut it short, employing the methods of wincing, shuddering, or a repelling chant to do so. And as soon as he abridges his memory of that event, and it ceases to occupy his mind, the reproach emotion fades with it almost instantly. In this way, he will proceed to cut short not just the memory, but any trains of thought that lead to the memory, and will also be extremely averse to remembering the event or discussing it in conversation. Eventually, both the event and its memory will become sequestered from his mind, and will only influence him as a minor annoyance in the rare times when something reminds him of it, and he has to invest a moment and a wince to deflect it.[29]

These features of the reproach emotion not only make it unlikely to be resolved by instinctive action, but render it largely inaccessible to conscious reappraisal as well. However, this doesn't normally pose much of a problem in a person's daily existence, since—unlike the emotions of sadness, anger, or anxiety, which extend beyond their instigating event and linger some time after they're evoked—the reproach emotion is tied solely to the memory of the event, and that memory remains almost completely cut off from the person's thoughts. We can therefore expect, in the absence of any competing factors, that a person will largely succeed in avoiding all his reproachful memories, and restrict the times he must feel the reproach emotion to the rare instances something reminds him of

---

[29] So effectively can a shameful event be blocked off from a person's mind, that the person will frequently forget, for long spans of time, that such an event ever occurred to him. He will sincerely respond in social situations, or on surveys, that he had never experienced any event like that, and will think of himself as somebody who something like that never happened to—even if it was earlier a central aspect of his self-image. When he is, however, directly confronted with remembering it (let's say by a friend who saw it take place), he will—almost invariably—openly acknowledge the event, and recognize it as something he always knew to have happened.

one.[30] But because the reproach emotion is so psychologically painful, and its influence on human behavior so self-destructive, it can
give rise to severe mental pathology if, compelled by an equally powerful motivation, the person becomes unable to flee from his shameful memories for any serious period of time. That is, as we'll shortly
see, exactly what happens in depression.

---

[30] But while one's memory of a shameful event only rarely evokes the reproach emotion, the influence a major event of this nature will have on a
person's future behavior is often enormous. It's usually the case, if the reproachful event was incurred in a meaningful area of the person's life, that
the person goes on to become overly defensive against recommitting the
same folly in future scenarios. This role is taken over by an unreasonably
intense emotion of anxiety, which emanates from similar situations where
the danger of repeating his past mistake lurks.
    Indeed, this seems to merely be an exaggerated reaction that is, in
its essence, the negative component of one and the same built-in imperative of the reproach emotion: to, next time, choose the correct course of
action in this type of scenario. It's interesting to observe that this negative
component is what gets retained, while the positive one is quick to disappear. More astounding is the paradoxical effect this quirk comes to have
on a person's behavior in situations similar to the past one in which he
incurred a severe reproach. In seeking this kind of situation, whether by his
original motivation to redo it or for some alternative reason, the person
finds himself wishing to recreate it, and simultaneously fearing it will turn
out the same way as the last. His resultant behavior is an odd compromise,
in which he approaches the situation with defensive caution, usually in sly,
backwards ways, attempting at the same time to achieve the result he desires, while excessively shielding himself from a reoccurrence of the shameful outcome he fears.
    This kind of behavior is almost always maladaptive. And it gives
us a powerful impression that the reproach emotion serves, above all, a
deep-seated learning function. It really appears to generate learning in two
different ways. In the first place, it teaches the person how not to behave
in a particular situation; and in the second place, although it rarely leads to
any positive action in the form of a successful redo, by urging the person
to play the scenario out in his fantasies, it leads him to think through the
correct way to act when a similar situation arises, which can eventually
prove useful, even if it only presents itself several years later.

The Psychology of Assigning Blame

Now that we are familiar with the reproach emotion, we can proceed to examine its critical role in depression. There is, however, another important topic I wish to touch upon first, which will provide a useful foundation for our upcoming analysis. It is a person's instinctual yearning for meaning, for reason.

In virtually every part of his life, but most strongly in events of great emotional significance, a person is compelled to seek a conscious understanding of it, to find the reason (or reasons) behind it. As part of this search for meaning, one indispensable question he gropes for an answer to is that of cause and effect. Whenever he experiences a displeasurable event, the person wants to know what caused it: what (or who) is responsible. But often, at least temporarily, he is unable to satisfy this desire by rational cognition, and this instinctual striving to link cause to effect is accomplished instead by subconsciously assigning blame.

For the unconscious mind, there exist only three ways to assign blame. A person either can blame himself, blame someone (or something) other than himself, or blame pure chance, probability, or fate—in essence, blaming nothing at all. Each of these three roads of blame leads to its own emotional reaction.

We already know that the first two (blaming yourself and blaming somebody else) each correspond directly to a specific emotion, and are a key element of the context needed to evoke it. Blaming yourself for an incurred displeasure, of course, is the primary factor that causes reproach emotion; and blaming your displeasure on somebody else is the exact evaluation that evokes anger. The third path, blaming your displeasure on chance, leads instead to liberation from emotion: the absence or negation of an emotional response. (I will discuss this third option later.)

For now, let us simply note the intriguing relationship between the emotions of anger and reproach. In a major respect, they can be considered polar opposites of each other: anger being the result of blaming displeasure on something external to you, and shame being the result of blaming it on yourself. Their effects are very similar, too: In anger, a person will seek to punish and get revenge on the target of his anger; and in reproach, the person will feel highly compelled to incur some punishment himself (at least in the verbal abuses he will direct at himself when experiencing the emotion). We also know that the same provoking event can lead alternately to anger or to shame. And it isn't uncommon that a person will vacillate between the two, having anger supplant shame and vice versa, as he tries to fit different interpretations to the event.[31]

What Happens Before Blame

In addition to these three roads of assigning blame, there is a fourth possibility: the main road that branches out into these three. It is the state in which a person has not yet decided who or what to blame: when he's unable to determine whether the blame for an event lies with himself, with somebody else, or if it's merely the result of pure chance. And this fourth scenario must, of course, precede any casting of blame, since it is the default condition that exists before blame is assigned.

---

[31] We should not make the mistake of thinking, however, that these are just two different sides of the same emotion. Anger and shame feel nothing alike, and their physiological effects are entirely different as well.

There are, however, instances in which a person feels *actual* anger at himself, at his own person. But this shouldn't be too surprising. Since people are able to view themselves, and their own actions, from an external perspective—and not exclusively from inside their own skin—it makes perfect sense that they would feel anger at themselves, exactly as they could at a third party, during those times when they *view* themselves as a third party. But this self-directed anger, in nearly all cases, is only a transient emotional state—only experienced while the person still casts about for an explanation behind some detrimental event, still tries to determine who is to blame, and what his own role in it really was. A person cannot remain angry at himself, or hold a grudge toward himself, or seek revenge over himself; while one's reproach emotion over a past misdeed most certainly can, and frequently does, last a lifetime.

The reason we went on this tangent to examine the process of blame is because it often is also a process of reevaluation. As we observed earlier, the reproach emotion is often evoked from a reevaluation of a displeasurable event—the reevaluation being that one personally caused that event (that one is to blame for it)—and as a result, the reproach emotion replaces, or at least supplements, another emotion that the event initially triggered. This exact same process, of course, can occur with anger as well. And this perfectly accords with our knowledge that, in the time before a person assigns blame for an event, what he most often experiences from it is a different negative emotion. (And the emotion must invariably be a negative and unpleasant one, if it is to ever evoke anger or shame.) Indeed, it's often precisely because some event triggered a strong negative emotion, that a person is compelled to assign blame for it.

The part of human psychology that makes this kind of blame and the emotions it evokes (either anger or shame) possible, is that the unconscious mind doesn't discriminate between types of displeasure. It doesn't matter whether the displeasure arises from a physical injury, a dissonant sound, a negative emotion, or a biological affect such as illness or hunger; the unconscious mind only registers that it is unpleasurable, and is thus free to employ any of them as the substrate for evoking an emotion. Thus, we arrive at the undeniable fact that one negative emotion can actually set off another—especially one of the blame emotions.

All of us probably know how quickly and easily a brief sadness caused by something trivial, such as spilling milk, is turned to anger if there is someone who can be blamed—for instance, a roommate who left the carton of milk on a precarious shelf in the fridge. So can the displeasurable affects of embarrassment, anxiety, and disgust be the cause of anger—for example, when a friend reveals an embarrassing story about you to others, or obliges you to attend an event that makes you nervous, or if you find yourself in a filthy environment you think was created by your friend's negligence. And each of these situations, we can be sure, can also evoke the reproach emotion, if we resolve to blame ourselves for it—such as concluding that it was our own clumsy behavior that spilled the milk, or exposed ourselves to embarrassment, and so on. On the other hand, if a person is unable to assign blame for such events (he refrains from doing so, or he cannot draw a conclusion as to the responsible party), no reevaluation occurs; and the original emotions of sadness, embarrassment, anxiety, disgust, and so on, remain as they were. And if the displeasure for which we don't assign blame is merely physical, such as stubbing one's toe on a table leg, that pain will evoke *no* emotion (in contrast to the anger it would arouse if we blamed a roommate for placing that table in a hazardous location).

Blameless Occurrences

Let us now turn to the last remaining alternative of blame, when a person recognizes that blame lies with pure chance, and that the event resulted from random and unforeseeable forces in the universe. This method of blame is especially unique. Unlike the other three paths of assigning blame, this one almost always requires a substantial amount of rational thought, knowledge, and conscious effort. Whereas linking an unpleasant event to something external, or to your own behavior, or not being able to make a link at all, requires practically no rational thought, and is in most cases accomplished completely subconsciously; for a person to truly recognize that an event is the result of chance, he must have a real conscious understanding of the chance forces that did cause it. It is precisely this understanding, and his awareness of the various chance circumstances leading up to an event, that separates one person's certainty that it is the result of fate, from another's uncertainty as to what caused it.[32]

---

[32] That assigning blame—to ourselves, or somebody else, or being unable to—is primarily an unconscious process, is shown by the fact that lower animals (who don't possess conscious thinking) are capable of all these reactions too. Dogs are certainly able to feel anger and shame—as shown by their bodies: tense, barking, and snarling when something angers them; and drooped ears, bowed head, and guilty eyes when they do something they

Blaming an event on chance is most certainly a reevaluation. In doing so, a person truly accomplishes a different framing of it in his mind. It ceases to be merely an event sprung upon him with no rhyme or reason, and becomes recognized as the product of some definite physical causes—which is, after all, the reevaluating effect of all manner of assigning blame. And this will remain, like all attributions of blame, an inseparable piece of information from the person's later memory of the event itself.[33] The effect of such a reevaluation on a negative emotional event is, normally, the highly beneficial one of ridding it of its emotional stigma.

While discerning that blame for an event lies only with fate may not have any effect in cases where the original source of displeasure is still present—such as an impending situation that causes anxiety, or a putrid object that causes disgust, or the consequences of a loss causing sadness, or even a nagging physical pain—it has a definite curative effect once that instigating factor has disappeared, and all that remains is the event's memory. It essentially closes the book on an event, resolving that it couldn't have been prevented, and that there's nothing further that can be done about it.[34] We may notice that in the resolution of grief after the death of a parent, as we mentioned earlier, precisely this type of reassessment that the death was a natural and unavoidable occurrence is what most commonly, and beneficially, takes place.

This type of conscious discernment of the random forces behind an event is a perfect example of the corrective, curative influence that rational reevaluation can have on emotional memories; and

---

know their owner doesn't approve of. They're also capable of reacting with neither of these emotions in response to an unpleasant stimulus. And there is no doubt that a large amount of their learning and functioning is determined by the way they draw causal links from unpleasant events.

[33] Occasionally, however, this kind of causal information *can* be forgotten (while the memory of the event remains intact), especially after long periods of time.

[34] It shouldn't surprise us, then, that such a perspective absolves an event of much of its emotional significance, since every negative emotion is by its nature a call to action.

it is a testament of the general therapeutic power of our conscious, rational mind, over our unconscious, emotional one. It is, in fact, very common that a struggle will play out in a person's mind between the subconscious impulse to cast blame on the first fitting target, and his rational analysis of the situation, which points to it being a blameless and chance occurrence.[35]

In *Figure 2* below, we can see the four general paths of blame a person can take in trying to identify the cause of an unpleasant occurrence. He will either (1) blame something external to him, and experience anger, (2) blame himself, and experience the reproach emotion, (3) blame fate or chance, and experience no emotions, or (4) be unable to determine where the blame lies, and be stuck with the original affect of the experience.

---

[35] A person will be compelled to instinctively cast blame, and will frequently experience short instances of anger and shame, in the course of rationally analyzing a situation and eventually coming to the conclusion that it was, in fact, the result of unforeseeable and uncontrollable chance.

For example, a person painfully bumping his head on a shelf or his foot on a chair may have an instantaneous reaction of irrational anger, even at an inanimate object or uninvolved person before realizing his own irrationality. So can a person feel an instant tinge of reproach after dropping and breaking some fragile glass object, before coming to his senses and recognizing that it was an accident. And most distinctively, a person gambling on a game of pure chance will often viscerally experience both anger and self-reproach after an unfavorable roll of the dice or turn of the card (anger at the dealer or some person he deems to be a source of bad luck, or reproach at himself for throwing the dice clumsily, and so on): events that by all tenets of reason are undeniably random.

The Four Roads of Assigning Blame

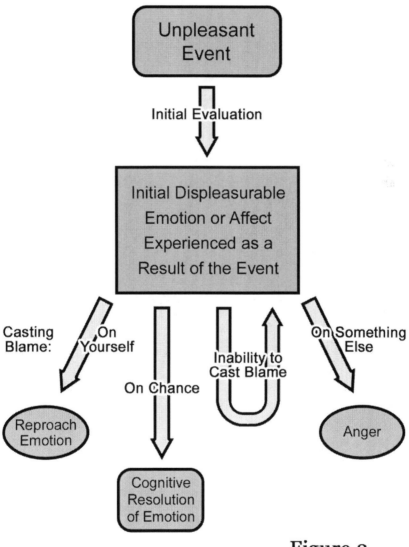

Figure 2

Individual Differences in Assigning Blame

Interestingly, as a consequence of explicit learning, past experiences, and genetic disposition, different people will have different patterns and habits of assigning blame. Thus, four individuals exposed to the same situation may each cast blame in a different way, and each have a different emotional response.[36]

Some people impulsively blame themselves at almost every opportunity (this is a common feature of many pathologies, especially depression). Some people compulsively blame others for any incurred inconvenience (this is a central feature of paranoia). In these cases, it is (1) unconscious evaluations transferred from prior experiences, (2) implicit beliefs about the self, the external world, and other people, and (3) one's immediate mood-state that are the factors chiefly responsible.[37]

There are people, too, who blame nearly all things on chance, fate, or accident (or, if religiously inclined, on God's will). And there are people who, in virtually all situations, choose to forego causal judgment, or are sincerely uncertain about where the blame lies. In these cases, it is (1) rational thinking, (2) explicit knowledge or

---

[36] That situation, however, must be ambiguous, where it is not automatically clear who or what is at fault. For instance, when it is clear that some harm is done to you by the deliberate and malevolent intention of another person, the situation is not open to various interpretations or the four alternatives of blame, and will invariably (at least at first) evoke anger.

[37] The effect of immediate mood-state shouldn't be underestimated. We know how a person already in an angry or irritated mood will find himself instantly, most often irrationally, and almost uncontrollably reacting with anger in situations he would normally consider innocent—and a person already feeling ashamed and reproachful will go on blaming himself for events that he otherwise never would. Moods and emotions alter cognition. And we can ourselves get a small glimpse of what is, for some people, a permanent state of depression or paranoia, when we ourselves experience their emotions and suddenly find our reality acquiring a new tint, and our perceptions and judgments being filtered through it.

beliefs, and (3) one's predominant mental state that are the factors chiefly responsible.[38]

Most people, however, will have different patterns and habits of assigning blame in different parts of their lives, and for different types of scenarios. A person, for instance, may typically react with anger whenever someone tells an embarrassing story about him, cast blame on himself and experience shame when he feels anxious about attending a party, recognize it as a chance occurrence when he is rejected by a girl, but be uncertain about what's responsible for him losing at blackjack.

Even so, all these are only general habits of assigning blame, and every individual can—at least occasionally—respond in ways contrary to his usual habits, depending primarily on his state of mind (the mood he is in, and his level of clarity or tiredness). In any case, it is clear that a person's usual habits of blame will have a massive effect on his daily behavior and personality.

The Drive to Cast Blame

One last thing I want to emphasize, before we move on from blame and back to depression, is how strikingly powerful the human urge to link cause to effect is. People will, after all, incur massive amounts of mental distress, by means of the blame emotions of anger and shame, merely to satisfy it. It thus supersedes our most basic instinctual drive to minimize and/or avoid displeasure.

---

[38] Because these are conclusions that must be reached consciously—either by recognizing the myriad of chance factors that caused an event, or failing to reach a decisive conclusion as to what caused it—they depend on a person's ability to think clearly, which in turn depends on his mental state (including his mood, his level of tiredness or alertness, and even his degree of intoxication). They also depend on his explicit knowledge—such as his knowledge that the way cards are dealt, or the way lottery numbers are chosen, is an entirely random process—which lets him better identify the chance causes behind some event.

Indeed, it runs completely contrary to the pleasure principle (the universal human striving to increase pleasure and reduce displeasure) that a slight and rather benign emotion of sadness—which a person experiences, for instance, from dropping a plate of food he looked forward to eating—would be replaced or conjoined with a fierce, fiery anger, or the especially painful reproach emotion, which clearly increases his overall level of displeasure, often acutely.[39] While this might not matter much—and have zero or few detrimental effects in the long run—when it comes to trivial situations like dropping a plate of food; this drive to cast blame, even at the expense of great mental distress, can wreak serious havoc when imposed upon major events in a person's life. We'll see a clear example of this in cases of depression.

---

[39] For an in-depth discussion of the pleasure principle, see my book: *Addiction, Procrastination, and Laziness: A Proactive Guide to the Psychology of Motivation*

Chapter 8

The Immature Romance:
An Analysis of One Type of Depression

Having explored the key psychological forces involved in depression, let's now investigate how they play out in the minds of depressed people. For this, we will examine one specific type of depression, one often observed by psychologists and laymen alike, and one I have experienced personally: the depression produced by the breakup of a psychologically immature romance.

By "psychologically immature romance," I mean a romantic relationship in which at least one of the partners is either an adolescent undistinguished for his or her psychological wisdom, or an adult who still retains many immature character traits of a typical adolescent. And though this is a somewhat garden-variety scenario, I have selected it here as our example because for this type of depression the causes, the mental processes that occur during the illness, and the ways it can be cured or overcome have all become known to me through introspection. I trust, therefore, that it will prove highly instructive.

To start, let us take note of the typical features most commonly present in these relationships. The renowned humanistic psychologist Abraham Maslow observed that these relationships weren't especially loving, warm, or affectionate, and were commonly full of deceit, insecurities, and a love-hate ambivalence. They were founded, he said, much less on a love, admiration, or fondness for the other person, and much more on that person's utility for satisfying one's own selfish needs and desires. In these cases, the partner was less of a lover and more of an object, a means more than an end. (Yet strangely enough, it is the loss of this type of unloving, immature romance that frequently leads to depression, while the loss of a loving, mature one more frequently leads to a regular grief.)

Maslow identified two basic elements of the immature romance: dependence and replaceability. In the relationships that culminate in depression, we consistently find both. Dependence refers to a state in which the satisfaction of one partner's basic psychological needs is provided solely by the other—something that extends far beyond just the physical sexual need. This aspect is nearly always true of at least one partner in a relationship that ends in depression—and specifically of the partner in whom the depression develops.

Replaceability refers to a person's ease in transitioning from one romantic partner to another, and his or her relative lack of discrimination about whom he or she chooses as a replacement. It is of little consequence to this person who the actual partner she becomes romantically involved with is, just as long as that partner adequately fills the required role. And this element is largely intertwined with dependence, since the role that that partner must fill is precisely one of providing satisfaction for the person's specific psychological needs. What is important to someone in such a relationship is not the unique individual he or she is involved with, but the things that this person provides and the idea that he or she symbolizes.

"The adolescent girl needs admiration per se," writes Abraham Maslow, "it therefore makes little difference [to her] who supplies this admiration." "One admiration supplier is about as good as another," and "these need-gratifying persons are interchangeable." It is important to mention that it is precisely in persons unable to find a replacement for their broken up immature romance in whom these depressions usually develop.

And so, we seem to already have reached a conundrum. Why does the loss of a petty relationship of this kind so often lead to a poisonous depression, while the much greater loss of a meaningful, loving relationship, or the death of a beloved parent, lead far more frequently to a regular, healthy sadness? There are several reasons behind this, the first of which we'll discover by more closely examining the psychological needs these relationships really satisfy.

Maslow identified these as well, in his hierarchy of human needs. At this point, however, we can no longer avoid discussing the fundamental differences between women and men. Although the basic human needs both the male and female seek to fulfill through a relationship are the same, their expression varies greatly in each gender.

Basic Needs and Gender Differences

Both genders seek self-esteem, a need to think well of oneself, to have evidence of one's own worth and virtue. For a man, a girlfriend provides this in being a symbol of his conquest, a testament to his ability to attract and master the opposite sex. For a woman, a boyfriend is validation that she is desirable, that she is worthy of being cared for and looked after, that she is deserving of love.[40] And it isn't merely the categorical knowledge of the other person's existence that provides this self-esteem (although that certainly is a large factor): That feeling of self-worth is rekindled and re-experienced in each tender moment the couple spends together.[41]

---

[40] It is relevant that we so commonly see women declare in their self-abasement that they are incapable of being loved, when—after the loss of this type of self-esteem providing romance—they are plunged into depression.
[41] This is also experienced as happiness in such moments, which is no coincidence. There is a large overlap between situations that evoke happiness and those that increase people's self-esteem. The happiness emotion is triggered by wish-fulfillment, when a person obtains something that he desires, whether it's due to his own effort, a gift from somebody else, or pure luck. Self-esteem is gained when he personally achieves some desire, or overcomes a challenge or hardship: when he recognizes himself as being the

Both genders, of course, seek basic human connection, friend-ship, somebody to commiserate with them and care about them. For men this more strongly signifies a partner in activities, somebody to have fun with, to absolve them of being alone. For women it is more someone to talk to, to confide in, to find support in and perhaps rely on. Of the psychological needs a relationship can satisfy, this is clearly the greatest and most fundamental. It's not hard to see how ending a romantic relationship that was also a person's main or only source of friendship can have disastrous effects, specifically to the tune of depression (and such cases are by no means rare).

Both genders seek future prospects of enjoyment, something to look forward to, hopes for a bright and exciting future. These mostly take the form of plans for future activities, both social and sexual, no matter how obscure or well thought out. For a man these usually involve taking the girlfriend places, giving her gifts, surprising her, attending exotic events together. And a girlfriend truly does open the path up to enjoying many such activities: ones that would normally be dull and unsatisfying, but which gain lots in the way of excitement when an intimate, romantic aspect is involved. The same is true for the woman, only her role in such activities is usually more passive. She wants to be taken places, to receive gifts, and so on. The differ-ence in sexual roles is of course obvious, and analogous.

Another psychological need these relationships can satisfy, alt-hough it's of lesser importance, is obtaining the respect and esteem of one's peers. This is a lot more the case for men than for women, at least in American society. For a man (especially an adolescent), an attractive and desirable girlfriend goes a long way in providing this. Here it is precisely the categorical knowledge of her existence that does the job, and among adolescent boys the simple facts of having

---

cause of his wish-fulfillment. It's clear that many events that evoke happi-ness also provide self-esteem. And just as a person needs a constant re-plenishment of happiness if he's to avoid growing discontent, he must also have a constant source of self-esteem or his feelings of self-worth will grad-ually fade.

sex and losing one's virginity before his pals do is a huge status symbol worthy of envy.[42] In women, the correspondence between the respect of their peers and having a boyfriend is tenuous, although it does tend to receive increasing admiration with age.[43]

We should of course understand that these differences between genders are merely general trends we observe, and that in actual individuals there are countless examples going against these trends. It is in fact nearly always possible to observe some aspect of the feminine psychological disposition in each man and the masculine psychological disposition in each woman. There are also many relationships between males and females in which these roles are reversed. And there are infinite shades of gradation that can be found in between. In romantic relationships between two people of the same sex, psychological differences due to gender are of course moot. Even in those, however, we usually find that one partner takes on a primarily masculine role and the other a feminine. In any case, whether a person's psychological needs take on a more masculine or a more feminine proclivity, the underlying needs for companionship, intimacy, a sense of self-worth, esteem in the eyes of others, and hopes for a bright and exciting future are universal to all human beings.

Losing What's Most Important

With that, we've arrived at one major reason why the loss of an immature romance (in the absence of a replacement) leads much more frequently to depression than the death of a parent in adulthood or the loss of a mature romance. It turns out to be, not a smaller loss as we initially assumed, but a decidedly greater one.

---

[42] And failing to do so often plays a very large role in adolescent depression in males.

[43] In adolescent depression in females, it's precisely the opposite factor of having lost one's virginity that is so often a large contributor (or at least that's what we find in American society, which is at least partially due to a cultural stigma).

A man who loses his mother may lose with her a large element of his life, but it's usually not one of crucial importance to his psychological health.[44] But a man whose plans and positive expectations of the future all involve or depend upon having a girlfriend (not at all an uncommon scenario, by the way) loses with her his whole optimistic outlook on the future—an utter loss of hope if he is unable to find a replacement.[45] The subjective loss of the latter man is certainly greater, even if he never cared much for the girl in the first place—it is his idea of her, and what she stood for in his mind, that he loses.[46]

For this same reason, the loss of a psychologically immature romance is greater than the loss of a psychologically mature one. After all, a big thing that makes a relationship psychologically immature is that it serves as the main or sole satisfaction of one or both partners' basic human needs. It is a psychological crutch of a sort, a literal dependence. In contrast, a mature relationship comprised of two psychologically healthy persons can practically be defined by the fact that it is not indispensable to the psychological

---

[44] This is different in the case of young children, for whom a parent (or parental figure) is all but a psychological necessity. It is understandable, then, why the death of a parent in childhood is such a strong predictor of future depression, and why it turns up so often in the history of people who describe themselves as having been depressed for their whole lives or "for as long as I can remember."

[45] His hopes then naturally shift to finding another girl to fill the vacant role in his imagination of the future, and we can ourselves imagine the bouts of discouragement this person will experience if he starts to doubt whether he'll ever be able to do so.

[46] Quite often, an adolescent who will experience depression after his immature breakup will also announce and even brag during the course of the romance that the girl he is dating means nothing to him, that he would readily replace her with someone better, and that he's emotionally detached from the relationship on the whole. (This was, indeed, precisely what happened in my case.) And in this, he will likely be telling the truth, at least as he sees it. What he doesn't realize is how much of his emotional pomp is derived from the mere fact of having this girlfriend. And he has no way of knowing how rapidly that bravado will disappear the moment its source is withdrawn from him.

wellbeing of either partner. Both partners have a stable sense of self-worth derived from sources unrelated to their relationship, they have other good friends and confidants besides their partner, their positive expectations for the future consist of more than just those involving a significant other, and their esteem in the eyes of their peers doesn't hinge on the existence of their romantic relationships (or they have grown past seeking it altogether).[47] For this type of person, the end of even a truly significant and loving relationship is only a partial loss that leaves him with much to fall back on.[48] But for a person who derived one or more of his basic need satisfactions exclusively from the relationship, its end (and continued absence) will be a lot more devastating—more like a total loss.

In this we can also recognize the roots of the depressed person's anhedonia, which isn't a feature of regular sadness. A person who experiences regular grief after the death of a parent or the breakup of a mature romance does not normally lose the capacity to enjoy himself or derive pleasure from his habitual sources, even though sadness likely discourages him from pursuing this. A depressed person, however, is characteristically taken by a complete or a partial anhedonia, and even his formerly favorite activities commonly cease to provide pleasure or hold any interest for him. We can finally see why: The first person's loss is not greatly related to the other important and enjoyable aspects of his life, while a person deprived of a dependent relationship loses the most important thing to him, his greatest source of esteem and enjoyment, next to which all other things pale in comparison and don't provide him with what he really wants.[49] This brings to mind a highly pertinent passage from Ayn

---

[47] It is this type of stability, and having various, consistent sources that satisfy one's basic human needs that contributes so much to a person's psychological health.

[48] This doesn't mean such a breakup is incapable of causing depression: it certainly is. It is simply less likely to do so.

[49] And this sheds light on another peculiarity of depression I mentioned briefly at the beginning of this book. It's that the anhedonic depressed person will usually have one particular type of activity or topic that he doesn't

Rand's *Atlas Shrugged*: "When nothing seems worth the effort . . . it's [only] a screen to hide a wish that's worth too much."

We should not make the mistake of assuming, however, that since psychologically immature, dependent relationships are so vital, and provide so much more for the persons involved, that they are also more nurturing, compassionate, and loving. Instead, they are the exact opposite. It is precisely this factor of dependence that is responsible for nearly all the malaise, dysfunction, relationship politics, and lovers' quarrels that occur in these romances—the normal result of conflicting interests between two needy, insecure people. And as we already mentioned, the actual interpersonal relations of these couples are not very warm or loving, but petty and scornful, since their relationships are based upon vain, narrowly selfish foundations, in which the partner is viewed less as a person and more as an object, primarily valuable in that he or she plays the set role of girlfriend or boyfriend.[50]

Inhibited Thinking

We've now identified one reason why these immature romances are so prone to ending in depression. Their loss, contrary to the way it first seemed, can reach devastating proportions. But this certainly isn't the most important factor. Even in the face of a huge, life-shattering loss, people are astoundingly resilient: They persist, they cope, they adapt, they reevaluate, and they recover. It is because we humans are endowed with a powerful set of mental faculties for rational

---

react to in his usual, uninterested way: a gap in his anhedonia. In this scenario, the content of the gap is entirely clear: It is any topic related to, or any activity that may hold the promise of, a new romantic relationship.

[50] In contrast, as a relationship approaches nearer and nearer to psychological maturity, health, and self-actualizing love, this aspect of role-playing gradually disappears, and with it so do the differentiated psychological proclivities of each gender. What remains at the end are two equal individuals, their differences determined much less by whether they're male or female, and much more by their unique individuality.

and analytic thinking, that we are able to deal with changes, to shift our goals, to intelligently pursue the satisfaction of our needs, and to overcome losses no matter how devastating.

In human beings, it is our conscious mind that is our most important tool for survival, and it truly is capable of amazing feats. In cases of loss such as the ones we just listed, the emotion of sadness has a very important biologically designated role in helping our rational minds adapt to the new circumstances. It has the effect of impelling us to focus all our cognitive efforts on that particular issue by rendering thoughts of anything else utterly uninteresting and unpleasurable. And that has a clear evolutionary advantage. It tells a person: "Stop! Do not proceed as planned. Withdraw for a time from the situation so you can reassess it, because a major change of a detrimental nature has most certainly just occurred. Think about what it means and how it affects you, because it might have just thrown all your past plans into shambles." This noble intention, however, is entirely thwarted when (as we know is so often the case in clinical depression) another factor exists to inhibit this conscious, analytical thought process from occurring.

What we find is that, in most cases of depression, and nearly always in those following the breakup of a psychologically immature romance, what inhibits the person's conscious analysis of his lost relationship (the same topic the emotion of sadness motivates him to dwell on) is the reproach emotion. To put it simply, this is a person who blames himself for having lost his relationship.

The Secret Inner Battle of the Depressed Mind

If we are to summarize the cognitive processes that generally take place in this person's mind, they would be the following:

(1) The person, having been deprived of a central part of his life, as well as a major source of enjoyment and satisfaction of his natural human needs, frequently pines to re-experience what he lost.

(2) This evokes the emotion of sadness and causes his thoughts to be drawn, as if for warmth, to memories of when he still possessed

what he now yearns for: the memories of his ended relationship. At this point the memories that appear in his mind are pleasurable, happy ones, and the reproach emotion is not yet evoked.

(3) But as he proceeds to think about and ruminate on his life situation as a whole, as the sadness emotion compels him to, that instant broadening of perspective promptly calls to his mind his overarching evaluation that all such happy moments are now lost, and that this is his own fault. (It is the memories of his own reproach-ful actions—actions that led, or that he thinks may have led, to the breakup—from which he initially drew that evaluation. And as his mind once again triggers that evaluation, those same memories are often recalled alongside it, at least on some unconscious level.)

(4) This then evokes a powerful reproach emotion, which causes the person to abandon and shrink away from any further thoughts on the subject. He may often do so with a self-chiding chant de-meaning his own person.

(5) This same cognitive routine will be repeated over and over again when the subject matter breaches his mind, preventing him from ever contemplating it long enough to fully work through it by conscious analysis and reason. (This is basically an emotional short-circuit, in which the actual aims of the emotion of sadness—to facil-itate conscious reevaluation and coping—are blocked off, leaving it the mere role of a painful dead weight that stubbornly resists the depressed person's attempt to move on and pulls him only further down into misery.) It will occur whenever the person is struck by a yearning for some particular enjoyment his relationship used to pro-vide, which will be often and unavoidable if—as is likely the case in this scenario—it was a basic human need.

(6) Each time this happens it will evoke a persisting bout of sad-ness, creating in the person the full clinical picture of depression. (This train of cognition will become increasingly automatic and un-conscious over time, often leading the person to forget or lose his awareness of where his depression originated in the first place.)

The Formula for Depression

We must pause here to fully absorb and appreciate this final point, because it is the central and most important one of this book. I will restate it: A person who (1) loses a romantic relationship that served as the sole satisfaction of one, or more, of his basic human needs, (2) blames himself for losing that relationship, and (3) fails to find a new relationship to replace it will already exhibit "the full clinical picture of depression."

I stated at the start of this inquiry that a core feature of depression is a persistent sadness that simply won't go away. The psychologist Seymour Epstein, acknowledging the same thing, observed that nearly all of the critical symptoms of major depression in the DSM can be fully accounted for by this "deep and enduring feeling of sadness." These symptoms are: (1) depressed mood; (2) diminished interest or pleasure in living; (3) fatigue or loss of energy; (4) motor agitation or lethargy; (5) diminished ability to think or concentrate (all of which are just the emotional, motivational, muscular, or cognitive symptoms of sadness); (6) increase or decrease in appetite, or else a significant weight loss or weight gain (the result of reduced pleasure in eating, in some people; or eating in order to soothe emotional stress, in others); (7) insomnia or hypersomnia (the emotional agitation of sadness preventing sleep—as all emotions have the potential for doing—in some people; or retreat into slumber to escape the pain of their sadness, in others); and (8) suicidal ideation or actual attempts at committing suicide (the depressed person's last and desperate solution to escape her emotional pain).

The only symptoms *not* accounted for by this emotion of sadness are (1) anhedonia, which is a mandatory part of depression, but isn't a feature of regular sadness, and (2) excessive feelings of worthlessness or guilt, which is an optional part of depression, certainly present in the vast majority of cases, but not in all. (I will discuss the depressions in which self-blame isn't present later on in the book.) What does explain these two remaining symptoms, however, are the two other features of the immature breakup: (1)

that what the depressed person lost is—at least for the moment—the most important thing to him, and (2) that he also blames himself for that loss.

I wrote that conclusion back in 2013; and since then, I have found numerous confirmations of it in a surprising variety of psychological writings.

For instance, I was highly surprised to find one author call depression "the refusal of grief," and another who called it "incomplete mourning." Of course, one reason a person may refuse to grieve, and thereby leave his mourning process incomplete, is that he cuts his thinking about a loss short due to reproach emotion.

In fact, this dismissing of thoughts and/or memories due to reproach emotion is nothing other than a classic Freudian form of repression. Freud conceived this mechanism of repression as the result of a conflict between the person's ego (his actual thoughts, actions, and desires) and his superego (the entire network of his moral ideas: consisting primarily of a strict set of moral commandments, acquired directly from his parents or other authority figures, as well as his moral ideal of what a good person should be like, acquired from the same source). When his actual behavior, whether mental or physical, clashes with his morality, the superego—acting through the intermediary of his conscience—causes him self-reproach.

This is, in fact, a remarkably accurate description of what activates the reproach emotion—except that it's only a special case. We of course know the reproach emotion, rather than resulting solely from a breach of the Freudian superego, simply occurs from behaving some way that we wish we hadn't, and that caused us distress that we could've avoided. Obviously, one reason a person might wish that he hadn't behaved in a certain way, is that it conflicts with the moral code he learned from his parents. But in this, another quote from Ayn Rand's *Atlas Shrugged* captures the essence of the matter: "Man's reason is his moral faculty," not his superego. And while some men do, in fact, reason by means of categorical prescriptions they learned from authority figures, that certainly isn't the only option.

Still, the idea that depression was the result of a person repressing his reaction to a loss because it conflicted in some way with his superego, became widely accepted among Freudian psychologists up to the 1980s. They even went as far as concluding that since the superego didn't develop until around adolescence—a very valid psychological observation, by the way—children younger than age twelve, or so, were simply incapable of having depression.[51] Since then, psychologists found that even at an incredibly early age, children most certainly *are* capable of depression. And they're also perfectly capable of repression, as well as self-blame.

Repression, for its part, needs have nothing to do with a superego or even with the reproach emotion. Repression, at its most fundamental level, is just an established avoidance response to some unpleasant mental content. We have evolved to avoid danger, in the external world, by instantly linking unpleasant sensations—like hitting one's shin on a rock, pricking one's hand on a bush, or burning oneself on a frying pan—to the physical objects that caused them, and then instinctively retreating from and later avoiding those objects. This highly adaptive mechanism, however, is often transposed—just as unconsciously, but much less successfully—on our internal world. When we experience some distressing thought, memory, or fantasy, which makes us feel a painful emotion (like anxiety), an unpleasant instinct (like disgust), or just an inexpedient bodily response (like getting an erection, blushing, or breaking into tears), we instantly link that negative affect to the cognition that caused it, and then mentally suppress that cognition to escape the affect. This usually works, at least partially, in the short run—but can

---

[51] The observation, initially made by Freud, that children didn't develop a superego until about adolescence, was later borne out by the great French psychologist Jean Piaget. Piaget carefully studied the cognitive development of children as they grew older, and he showed that it wasn't until age eleven or twelve that the vast majority of children entered what he called the "formal operational" stage of mental development. Only at this stage did they become capable of fully explicit, abstract reasoning—which also included the abstract moral reasoning of the Freudian superego.

prove disastrous in the long run. When avoiding specific mental content (like memories of one's dead mother) becomes a habitual, long-term response, *that* is repression.

To put it another way: Repression is consistently treating particular thoughts, memories, or fantasies as though they were physical objects to be avoided. Reproach emotion due to a breach of one's superego is only one reason for this avoidance. There are certainly many others, and these can be present in young children as well. My girlfriend at the time of writing this, who had a difficult childhood filled with traumatic experiences that strongly portended a later depression, and who indeed went on to experience several severe episodes, described to me one such reason. Her divorced, temperamental, narcissistic mother would physically beat her since she was just two years old. If something the child did upset her, or if she had a frustrating day at work, she'd often fly into an unavoidable, unpredictable rage, grab hold of the nearest suitable object (be it a belt, coat hanger, or frying pan), and use it to hit her cowering daughter over the limbs, body, and head, until her fury was fully spent. If the daughter showed fear, anger, or broke into tears, the mother would threaten "I'll give you something to really cry about," and then beat the girl harder unless she stopped. My girlfriend soon learned to repress her emotions to avoid these intensified beatings. In her household, repression became a matter of course.

Self-blame, too, is undoubtedly possible to young children, and it is plainly observable in kids ages four or five. Seymour Epstein notes, quite remarkably, that kids of abusive parents—and often the ones who later experience depression—commonly blame that abuse on themselves, since viewing themselves as "bad" and the parent as "good" is less distressing for them than thinking the opposite. Having evolved to seek out their parents' love and acceptance (on which their survival and flourishing depends), this leaves them the hope of changing themselves to become "good," by their parent's standard, and thereby achieve that objective. Other writers on depression affirmed this to be their experience, and so has my present girlfriend. Richard O'Connor was right in viewing repression and self-blame as two of the many "skills" a person can learn in his early life that then predispose him to getting depression.[52]

---

[52] Despite its obvious shortcomings, this view of depression as a repressed mourning puts it in an intriguing context. Other mental illnesses, like certain forms of Obsessive-Compulsive Disorder, operate in the same way.

In those instances, it's often some sexual impulse or desire that gets repressed: A person (an adolescent or psychologically immature grownup) experiences some sexual thoughts, feelings, or fantasies, which he rejects out of reproach, anxiety, or both, and therefore dismisses them from his mind any time they occur. Maybe it's sexual thoughts about his mother, or sister, or a member of the same sex. Maybe those sexual desires are deviant in some other way. Maybe his sexual fantasies are in fact normal, even socially acceptable (by adult standards), but appear alien, violent, and even insane to the adolescent possessed by them for the first time. Maybe he's terrified that his parents will learn and disown him, or his peers will find out and ostracize him, or that God's judging his thoughts and will cast him in hell for it. Maybe he's scared that he'll act on those impulses. Maybe his church taught him his sexual desires are evil. Maybe he fears he's becoming a depraved monster. Or maybe all the above.

In any case, because his sexual instincts can't be repressed, those very same thoughts, feelings, or fantasies will keep coming back (the obsession), and he'll need to mobilize some counterthought, chant, or behavioral ritual to force them away again (the compulsion). Alternately, in some other cases of Obsessive-Compulsive Disorder, it is the person's angry or violent thoughts, feelings, or fantasies—like a desire to kill his parents, children, or spouse—that get repressed, and for all the same reasons. And Freud himself described one famous case in which the violent and sexual desires were one and the same (see his "Case of the Ratman," in *The Wolfman and Other Cases*).

From this perspective, the malady of depression need not seem like such an anomaly to us. It after all follows, in at least some of its forms, the same basic principles of psychopathology as other common varieties of mental illness. The same way those cases of OCD are caused by the person repressing his vengeful or sexual desires, which obviously don't disappear since they are neither reevaluated nor acted upon, and which therefore persist as intrusive obsessional thoughts; so is depression, in some instances, caused by a person repressing his grieving response after a loss, which also won't go away, and therefore persists as a perpetually empty, depressed mood.

As for the anhedonia element of depression, I was surprised to find that here too my conclusion was mirrored by two (Neo-Analytic) psychologists: Silvano Arieti and Jules Bemporad. Severe depression, they wrote, is caused by "a loss of what seems to the patient the most valuable or meaningful aspect of his life," along with "the feeling of being unable to retrieve or substitute what has been lost."

Finally, my conclusion that, in many cases of depression, the person actually blames himself for the loss he incurred, was more than sufficiently verified for me by an abundance of different sources. "One of the chief risks of divorce," writes Richard O'Connor, "is that the child will blame himself," which also accounts for the remarkably high rates of depression among kids of divorced parents. Children of suicides, too, "often internalize blame" for their parents' deaths, observes Andrew Solomon, and their rates of depression are also abnormally high. One acute case, described by Aaron Beck, vividly illustrates a traumatic event that seems perfectly tailored to causing depression. An American soldier in the Korean war, while horsing around in the trenches with his best buddy Buck—"the only person who ever understood or loved me"—accidentally fired a loaded rifle into Buck's mouth and killed him. He was handed a three-year prison term for "culpable negligence," and developed a severe psychotic depression. His case was just one of five highly similar ones in which a soldier accidentally shot and killed a good friend, and all of which ended in a severe depression. Self-blame for the accident was explicitly reported in each case.

A recent memoir by the late mixed martial artist Josh Samman discloses another, very similar tragedy. He was texting his longtime girlfriend, his "best friend [and] soulmate," as she drove through a thunderstorm; and just minutes after he sent his last text, her car veered off the road and crashed into a tree, killing her. The exact cause of the accident couldn't be known, but Josh blamed himself—and fell into a morbid depression. "You killed the one you claimed to love most," was what he concluded.

The Self-Blaming Breakup

Having taken this brief detour to consolidate our gains, we'll now return to our original trail of inquiry (the depression produced by an immature breakup), since it still contains issues we haven't addressed yet.

Mainly, we have to ask: What is it about these immature romances that makes them so much more likely to end in a self-blaming breakup (as they most certainly are) than mature ones? Well, the answer to this can be found on two levels: First, in the psychology of the persons who make that evaluation; and second, in the conditions that reign in those relationships themselves.

Clearly, to reflexively blame oneself in ambiguous situations, and to not recognize those events to be accidents or inevitabilities when reassessing them consciously, is a hallmark of psychological immaturity—or poor psychological health.[53] The connection

---

[53] The terms 'psychological health' and 'psychological maturity or immaturity' can often refer to the same thing, but they are two distinct concepts. A person's psychological health refers to the overall levels of mental distress and wellbeing he experiences (averaged over a substantial period of time) from the way he reacts and relates to the world, to other people, and to his own mental processes. His psychological maturity or immaturity refers to his progress in gaining certain specific skills, understandings, and experiences that reduce mental distress and promote mental wellbeing, but which are normally absent during one's youth. Thus, a person's psychological maturity or immaturity is just one age-dependent dimension of his psychological health.

It isn't psychologically unhealthy, for example, for an adolescent to act like an adolescent—angsty, and needy, and sex-obsessed—but it is psychologically immature. Such behavior stems, after all, from not understanding his own mental functions (which takes time and effort, and which he's only just spawned the capacity to understand), and from the non-fulfillment of some basic human needs, like sex, respect, and self-esteem (which also take time and effort, and which he's just recently spawned the urge to fulfill). It is, however, both psychologically unhealthy and immature for an adult to behave like an adolescent. And it is neither mature nor immature, but clearly psychologically unhealthy, for either an adult or adolescent to have a full-blown mental illness, such as depression, phobias, or

between self-blame and the immature romance, therefore, may be that they're both caused by this third variable: the psychology of the immature or neurotic person, who not only forms this type of relationship, but is likely to blame himself when things go wrong.

This, however, can only partially account for the facts: because, on another level, there often are situational factors in an immature romance (or the way that it ends) that make it more conducive to a verdict of self-blame (or a verdict that resists reassessment) than a more mature one. In other words, the conditions that reign in the relationships themselves render them especially likely to terminate in enduring self-blame—whether or not the persons involved are psychologically predisposed to it. And on this level, we can readily recognize one feature of these relationships that makes their closing acts vulnerable to such an evaluation. It is that there's often a large measure of vagueness and loose ends to these breakups—an element of uncertainty commonly present within immature romances even while they last.

Uncertainty

Uncertainty, as I described earlier, prevents a person from conclusively deciding what caused a detrimental event, and resigns him to unconsciously assigning blame for it, leaving the road open to just the two blame emotions of anger and shame.

One reason an element of uncertainty is such a common feature of immature breakups is that the bonds holding the two partners together are not very strong in the first place. They often aren't especially fond of each other; there isn't a lot of empathy between them; they're prone to get into petty quarrels; and they frequently come to take their partner for granted, failing to realize how much psychological benefit they really derive from that person. Under

---

obsessive-compulsive disorder, since the conditions that cause these dysfunctions—like a certain traumatic experience—are not an inherent part of one's youth.

these conditions, a breakup may easily occur on a whim, or a misunderstanding, or an outburst of temper, with no great imperative for either partner to reconcile or even discuss it.

In this lies an important difference between this type of relationship and a psychologically mature one. In the latter, when the relationship ends, it's much more likely to be a decision reached by mutual consensus, or at least one partner's explicit disclosure as to why he or she wishes to break things off. That's partially due to a higher level of care and compassion between the two partners, so that neither, out of sympathy, would like leaving the other person in the lurch—or they would probably experience guilt and reproach for it. And it's partially due to their lives having, very likely, become more intertwined, making an upfront confrontation about their breakup much harder to avoid.[54]

Another huge factor that adds uncertainty to an immature breakup is that, even before the breakup, there's often only a dubious understanding between the two partners. They tend to be rather inhibited around each other; to communicate poorly, infrequently, or dishonestly; and therefore to stand on highly tenuous ground in regard to their partner—not really sure what they mean to the other person, what keeps them together, or what the other wants or expects of them. While in a mature romance, there's likely to be extensive discussion about such matters; in an immature romance, the partners are prone to hesitate, dread, or even fear inquiring into them. This kind of discussion, they often feel, can easily compromise the whole relationship, being unsure of their own personal

---

[54] It is vital to understand that relationships aren't, by way of dichotomy, either psychologically mature or immature; and if a relationship is one, then it certainly can't be the other. A totally mature and a totally immature relationship are opposite extremes, with an infinite range of gradations that lie in between them. All real relationships fall somewhere inside that range—containing some elements of psychological dependence and immaturity, and some elements of care, understanding, and healthy compassion. In actual life, psychological maturity and immaturity are always a matter of degree.

motivations, and doubly unsure about whether, if disclosed, those motivations would be acceptable to their partner. As a result, an immature breakup will frequently occur without one or both partners really knowing the reasons behind it—not fully sure about what they did wrong, or what they were doing right in the first place.[55]

It's these peculiar conditions in immature romances that tend to estrange the event of their loss from a person's conscious under-standing—and much more so than is normally the case in most other types of large losses. In most other scenarios where a person loses something of great value to him, including the death of a parent, we can expect the causes and details of the loss to be plainly evident—rather than shrouded in uncertainty, as we frequently find in these situations.[56] This uncertainty makes the person unable, in his psycho-logical compulsion to link cause to effect (which is especially strong

---

[55] After every such breakup, however, both partners will ravenously at-tempt to deduce—using logic and reason—the answer to all of these ques-tions about their relationship and the way it ended, forming elaborate theories based upon all the evidence they have. And yet these theories, however well-founded they may be, lack that distinct stamp of certainty and fact, which prevents a person from decisively pinpointing the cause of his breakup, and mostly resigns him to dubiously assigning blame.

[56] One massive exception to this is the suicide of a parent (or, for that matter, of a child or spouse). Even with a suicide note, and in most cases there isn't one, it's almost impossible to find out with certainty why a sui-cide victim ended his life. The person's no longer there to tell you his rea-sons and motivations, and all you can do is theorize and grasp at straws using whatever evidence you have, and likely reproach and blame yourself for any part you had played—or suspect you had played—in contributing to it. This makes a loved one's suicide a nearly perfect recipe for depres-sion. It is why suicides are often "contagious," with a loved one's suicide often precipitating depression and further suicides in those who survive him, and who not infrequently kill themselves in the exact same manner as their beloved. (See *The Noonday Demon*, Chapter 7.)

A parent's suicide is especially perilous to a young child, who's not only at a clear disadvantage in terms of consciously processing such a huge loss, but whose remaining caregivers—as John Bowlby pointed out—often take pains to hide the true details of the suicide from the child, leaving the

in highly emotional scenarios), to attribute the cause of his loss to chance or to fate, which greatly increases the likelihood of him blaming himself, and which greatly increases the likelihood of depression.[57]

But uncertainty alone, even without turning into self-blame, can itself be sufficient to inhibit the processing of a loss that can then lead to depression. After all, as Seymour Epstein points out, there are also depressions without feelings of worthlessness, self-hate, and self-blame. Depression, like grief, is a prolonged period of sadness, which only comes to an end once the person has processed his loss and achieved a reevaluation (or, in some cases of depression, found a replacement). Without persistent self-blame, which is a usual but not mandatory symptom, the one thing that differentiates depression from grief is anhedonia. And this, we know, is caused by the depressed person losing not just something valuable to him, but something supremely valuable to him, something he considers completely indispensable, and which he has no foreseeable hopes of replacing.

The mind is the chief mechanism by which human beings adapt to reality. Sadness facilitates this adaptation to the new reality we're faced with after a loss. (In grief, it's a partial loss; in depression, it's a total loss.) It does this by attracting our thoughts and attention to that loss, and will persist until we've adapted to it—either physically,

---

ghastly event shrouded in mystery, and frequently leading the child to blame himself. (See *Attachment and Loss, Volume 3,* Chapter 22.) Children of suicides, as we know, have extremely high rates of depression. And in the case histories of the most severe depressions, a parent's suicide is found surprisingly often.

[57] It isn't a pivotal factor, however, which one of the partners initiates the breakup. Whether a person withdraws from the relationship himself in response to some unpleasant event, or merely plays his own part in a conflict that causes his partner to do so, both provide ample grounds—since each played an active role in the episode—for a verdict of self-blame that can lead to depression.

As for whether depression develops in both partners, in just one, or in neither, all three have a fair probability. For either person to contract depression, it is simply a question of him or her meeting the needed psychological conditions.

by finding a replacement, or mentally, by reaching a reevaluation. But this process of adaptation can take multiple months or years—which is, correspondingly, how long one's depression or grief period will last. There can also be inhibiting factors, such as drugs, alcohol, and self-blame, which interfere with this process of adaptation, and therefore prolong it. Uncertainty, too, can play this same role.

A man who's unsure of what caused his loss—or, as sometimes happens, of what he lost—will be faced with a much more difficult, and therefore much lengthier, process of adaptation. For example: A man who can't find the reason his girlfriend broke up with him will have a much harder time coming to terms with and reevaluating his loss, because he can't even tell why it happened. Even without casting blame in either direction, as we can see in *Figure 2*, he'll still retain his original emotion of sadness, and (if his loss was a total one) remain stuck in a state of depression.[58] In cases like this, however, the

---

[58] In fact, this type of non-self-hating depression, sustained by uncertainty alone, appears to occur much more frequently in cases caused by the loss of some future prospect—a purpose, a goal, an aspiration, an expectation, a hope—than in the scenarios we're examining. In those cases, it's often by no means obvious exactly what has been lost, how it was lost, or what the person can do to replace it. And the very considerable challenge, in this type of depression, is simply figuring all this out, which on its own can take months or years, without any interference from self-blame.

The renowned 19th century Russian writer Leo Tolstoy suffered from this kind of depression, which struck him at age forty-nine, when—as he described it—"I had a good wife who loved me and whom I loved, good children, and a large estate . . . , was respected by my relations and acquaintances . . . , and without much self-deception could consider that my name was famous," when he suddenly found that "there were no wishes the fulfillment of which" he desired. In order to further build his estate, or educate his children, or write a book, he said, "I had to know *why* I was doing it." And without knowing why, "I could do nothing and could not live." While imagining growing his estate to 16,000 acres and 300 horses, "the question would suddenly occur . . . and what then?" "Or when considering plans for the education of my children, I would say to myself: 'What for?' Or when considering how the peasants might become prosperous, I would suddenly say to myself: 'But what does it matter to me?' Or

human compulsion to link cause to effect is so strong that the man
normally can't resist casting blame, on either himself or his ex-girlfriend, to avoid a state of total confusion—which truly is a lot less

---

when thinking of the fame my works would bring me, I would say to myself, 'Very well; you will be more famous than Gogol or Pushkin or Shake-
speare or Molière, or than all the writers in the world—and what of it?'"
And he found "no answer." He felt that everything "I had been standing
on had collapsed," and everything "I had lived on no longer existed." He
became swamped by a total anhedonia, an inability to act, and desires for
suicide, but no self-revulsion. He finally concluded "that life was meaningless," a question he would grapple with, depressively, to the end of his life.

The 19th century English philosopher John Stuart Mill suffered
from this kind of depression as well. Since his mid-adolescence, he wrote,
"I had what might truly be called an object in life; to be a reformer of the
world." And "my conception of my own happiness was entirely identified
with this object." Then, at age twenty, it somehow "occurred to me to put
the question directly to myself: 'Suppose that all your objects in life were
realized; that all the changes in institutions and opinions which you are
looking forward to, could be completely effected at this very instant: would
this be a great joy and happiness to you?' And an irrepressible self-con-
sciousness distinctly answered, 'No!' At this my heart sank within me: the
whole foundation on which my life was constructed fell down. All my happiness was to have been found in the continual pursuit of this end. The
end had ceased to charm, and how could there ever again be any interest
in the means? I seemed to have nothing left to live for." He too fell into
depression and anhedonia, but without any self-hatred. He, however, made
a full recovery.

The great 20th century fiction writer and philosopher Ayn Rand,
after finishing *Atlas Shrugged*—her last novel and magnum opus, on which
she labored for thirteen straight years—also fell into this type of depression. She had "a mission in life—and that was to write *Atlas Shrugged*."
Having finished and published the book, she expected that it would have
an instant, revolutionary effect on the world—which didn't transpire. Finding no new mission to devote herself to, and being profoundly disappointed at her book's lack of impact, she became anhedonic and depressed
(but without the self-hatred), which lasted for several years. This is, in fact,
a fairly common phenomenon among writers, often half-jokingly referred
to as post-publication depression. (See *My Confession*, by Leo Tolstoy, Chapters 3 and 4; *The Autobiography of John Stuart Mill*, by John Stuart Mill, Chapter 5; *Ayn Rand and the World She Made*, by Anne Heller, Chapter 13, and
Judgment Day: My Years with Ayn Rand, by Nathaniel Branden, page 218.)

bearable. In doing so, he'll grasp at any plausible basis, any feasible theory, to support a verdict of either reproach at himself or anger at his former partner—or, as actually happens quite often in cases of uncertainty, will vacillate between the emotions of anger and shame, while living with two (or more) competing theories of what really happened.

On top of that, the presence of uncertainty makes the person less likely to assign blame based on actual fact, merit, and evidence. The way he casts blame, in the absence of full information, will be more strongly determined by his proclivities and past experiences: the mental schemas by which he unconsciously frames events and allots blame (similar to how one projects his own personal preferences upon an ambiguous inkblot test). And since people who form immature relationships are more likely to be unconsciously self-blaming, this tips the scales even further in the direction of self-reproach.

But these unconscious schemas don't replace conscious thinking and reason, they merely bias it; they channel the person's explicit reasoning process to first arrive at and then maintain an emotionally compelling conclusion. In this, we're able to recognize two distinct threads of reproachful memories in the person who blames himself for an immature breakup: (1) his classically reproachful memories, of actions taken toward his former partner that he regretted even before the breakup, and which may have been used as initial evidence for his overall verdict of self-blame, and (2) his retroactively reproachful memories, of ambiguous actions he wasn't ashamed of before the breakup, but which he now reevaluates (in the fog of uncertainty) as having possibly contributed to it, thereby recruiting them as further confirmation—as rationalizations—for the self-blaming conclusion already arrived at by unconscious, emotional means. Although this first thread of memories constitutes nothing abnormal, and can be found in the history of almost any relationship; it is this second thread of reproachful memories, which can proliferate wildly when bred in uncertainty, that sets off—in most cases—the raging torrent of abuse, disparagement, and reproaches the melancholic directs at himself.[59]

---

[59] This last point is worth emphasizing: Being assailed with reproachful memories in the wake of a large loss isn't exclusively a feature of depression. It can be, and often is, also a feature of healthy mourning.

By sheer virtue of time, throughout the history of almost any relationship—be it mature or immature, romantic or casual, parental or filial—there's bound to be some amount of reproachful memories peppered in with the rest. And when that relationship ends, like after the death of a parent, these memories form a substantial part of the total memories the person must revisit, reassess, and make peace with in the course of his grieving process.

There's also a third thread of reproachful memories, essentially independent of the first two, that only becomes reproachful once the loss has occurred—the clear result of a reevaluation. This is the normal regret that frequently emerges after a major death (and which greatly contributes to how large of a loss that death is). Usually, a person has many memories of unsatisfying interactions with a loved one that don't bother him, have no real bearing on everyday life, and are practically never thought about or forgotten—as long as that loved one still lives. But after his or her death, these memories undergo a reevaluation, and come back—even in the course of healthy bereavement—in the form of painful regrets and reproaches.

Fundamentally, people love booking wins. And they hate notching a loss or suboptimal transaction. When they get ripped off on a purchase, even for a petty amount of money, they'll often fume, torment themselves, and feel self-reproach over it for days, weeks, and sometimes months after it happens. When playing the stock market, they tend to sell out of their winning positions and hold on to their losing ones, notching a win in the former while not accepting a loss in the latter, even though this amounts to keeping their losing stocks and dumping their winners, which loses them money in the long run. (See *Thinking, Fast and Slow,* by Daniel Kahneman, page 214.)

The death of a loved one is very much like that: It is an involuntary closing of a position, whether you were up on that position or down, whether you made the most of your time with that person or you didn't. Once death has come, it's over, the account is closed; and if the surviving person didn't get all he wanted from that relationship—he never told his dead father something he wished to, or never asked him some crucial question, or never received some response he had yearned for—he'll likely experience the same basic buyer's remorse as the man who got ripped off buying a used car, and go through all the same torments, regrets, and

The human mind, however, does not simply take all this lying down. It isn't content to live with uncertainty, even when blame is assigned. The person experiences this type of uncertainty as its own distinct kind of displeasure. He knows, at least on some unconscious level, that casting blame is but an inadequate substitute for what he really wants: factual knowledge, to find out exactly why the breakup occurred, and to attain certainty. The person will seek this information vigorously, he will yearn for it, but he might go his whole life without finding it. In psychological parlance, this is astutely acknowledged as the need for closure—the therapeutic effects of which we'll discuss shortly.

Closure as a Cure for Uncertainly

We've thus reached a rather satisfying explanation for why the breakup of an immature romance so frequently leads to depression. It combines a massive loss with a large element of uncertainty, which is either sufficient all on its own, or potentiates a conclusion of self-blame, to prevent the loss from being worked over by conscious reappraisal. But uncertainty, from what we know about casting blame, isn't a necessary element in the formula for depression. The same essential conditions can be, and frequently are, met when a person

---

kicking himself in the course of his grieving process. This is another non-pathological type of reproach that only makes itself felt after a loved one's death, but which remains dormant and untroubling while that person is still alive—because, at that point, the position is still open, the loss hasn't been notched yet, and there still remains time to make amends.

All this, of course, is very different from actually blaming oneself for a loved one's death, which shrouds the whole lost relationship in the shadow of self-reproach, instead of certain specific parts of it. Only *that* cuts the whole subject of the loss off from conscious analysis. And only that, especially when combined with uncertainty, appears to be a sure formula for depression.

knows for certain the true cause of his breakup, and that that cause was his own behavior.[60]

Still, self-reproach combined with uncertainty tends to result in a much more tenacious depression than just uncertainty or self-blame alone. Naked uncertainty, without self-blame, can be resolved by explicitly identifying what has transpired: a much easier process with no reproach emotion to stand in the way and make the person repress the thoughts and memories most needed to do so. Legitimate self-blame, in which a person knows for a fact that he is the cause of his own major loss, can be resolved by thoroughly understanding and coming to terms with the actions that caused it: seeing that they were the inevitable result of his beliefs, psychological state, and circumstances at the time. This is a powerful insight and truly curative reassessment, in which a person transcends his narrow view of himself as an actor, and thereby frees himself from his self-reproach, by recognizing that even his own actions were the fated result of forces outside his control. The presence of uncertainty, however, will make a person incapable of achieving this insight, since he won't even know exactly which actions he must come to terms with. And here we can recognize one major benefit of closure.

Closure is obtaining conclusive information about an event that eliminates the uncertainty around it, and enables the person to place a decisive interpretation on it. It's often highly therapeutic, and is a critical staple in many approaches to psychotherapy, including some targeting depression. We can certainly see, in our example of the immature breakup, what profound benefits it can have: Obtaining closure might let a person discover that his breakup was inevitable, out of anybody's control, which instantly opens the path to overcoming his depression. It may let him discover that the fault lies with his former partner instead, or with somebody else entirely, and this too

---

[60] We also know that, even in the presence of uncertainty, a person can cast blame in a totally different direction and evoke the emotion of anger instead. We've all surely heard of the vengeful breakup, which can be considered the polar opposite of the kind we're examining here.

will absolve him of self-reproach—and if not fully dispel his depression, then make consciously processing his loss a whole lot easier.[61] And even if the person discovers that he really was the one who's at fault, that still is a lot better than what existed before it, since he now has a chance to face up to the actual actions that led to the breakup, make peace with them, and achieve a reevaluation. In all permutations of depression combined with uncertainty, closure is decidedly beneficial and tips the scales greatly in favor of a healthy recovery.

Replaceability as an Obstacle to Closure

There is, however, one final factor in immature romances that works to prevent the pursuit of closure, which adds yet another reason why they so frequently end in depression. This is the element of replaceability in an immature romance. The main motivation of sadness, which a person experiences from losing his relationship, is to find a replacement for what he lost. Where there is uncertainty surrounding the breakup, that and closure are the two things he will seek. But while closure is best obtained from that ex-partner, replaceability pronounces her unimportant, and essentially steers the person to hunt for a replacement in anybody but her.

After all, he does not preferentially want that specific girl back, just about any girl will do (or at least one that meets his standards); and his ex-partner becomes an especially unattractive option, because of all the past issues he needs to confront and repair to regain her favor. He'd much rather get a fresh start with somebody new—and he is not wrong to want that.[62] Yet he fails to realize that,

---

[61] Although anger can still be a complicating factor, and a real distraction from processing a large loss, it simply doesn't produce the same magnitude of repression that self-reproach does. It's also a lot easier to forgive another person (to reevaluate anger) than to forgive oneself (to reevaluate shame)—and it certainly happens a lot more often.

[62] The situation is a very different one for the person getting out of a healthy, mature relationship. What she cared for and lost was a unique individual—important for his personality, his values, and his goals—and not

psychologically, it is his ex-partner who carries the key to overcoming his depression.

This blocks the most direct route to closure he has. And frequently, the self-reproach he associates with his ex-partner, and his dread of confronting it, will cause him to do whatever he can to avoid seeing her, meeting her, or speaking to her ever again.[63] Despite this, the person will continue to crave and pursue closure. Even as he completely avoids all confrontation with his ex-girlfriend, he will still try to find a definitive answer for what caused her to play her role in the breakup, only using covert, indirect, surreptitious means—which will probably prove unsuccessful.

Replaceability as a Misleading Belief

Adding to that, the replaceability factor can work to promote depression in yet another (purely cognitive) way. In those particular cases of depression where the person has attained closure and discovered for certain that he really was to blame for the breakup, considering his ex-partner unimportant may make him dismiss his own thoughts and reflections over the matter as unimportant as well, thereby neglecting to pursue them, and thus foregoing the cognitive work needed to reassess the whole episode.

---

mainly a stand-in who filled the set role of boyfriend. In her sadness, therefore, she isn't as willing to accept a replacement, even when she can easily find one. After all, a different person would not really help her regain what she lost. She could only do so by returning to that specific person, or otherwise finding someone very much like him.

[63] In this, we can recognize one more reason why an immature breakup is so conducive to causing depression. After all, this type of breakup—in which the two former partners never again see or speak to each other—is very much like a death. And just like a death, it often leaves a person with all sorts of unamended regrets—things left unsaid, questions left unasked, feelings left unexpressed, and desires left unfulfilled—which makes the magnitude of the loss so much greater. This is in very stark contrast to a mature breakup, which usually ends with the ex-partners remaining friends, or at least being on speaking terms, leaving the door open to say what was left unsaid, ask what was left unasked, and amend any past wrongs.

For this very same reason, the person who ends up depressed after an immature breakup will often be ignorant of what really caused his depression. He will refute the idea that it's the result of that ended relationship, because—by his standards—he truly didn't care much about the person he had it with. Or perhaps, in an alternate twist on this same theme, he may conclude (out of pride) that he *shouldn't* care much about the person he had it with, and thus refuse to accept the idea that his depression resulted from losing that person. (This is, in fact, a great example of the grieving response being repressed because it conflicts with a certain dimension of the Freudian superego—namely, pride.)

Chapter 9

My Personal Encounter with Depression

To crown our investigation, I now wish to share a firsthand account of my own episode of depression, which exhibited most of the psychological features we examined above.

One summer off from high school, when I was a sexually frustrated adolescent of age fifteen, I found my first girlfriend in a small rural hamlet in upstate New York. It was the summer dacha of my two grandparents, who invited me there for a few weeks to spend time with them, and to escape the blazing New York City heat, which my parents also urged me to do. I was rather fond of my grandparents, and most of my friends left for camp that summer, so I decided to accept their invitation, and relax there for an indefinite time until I grew tired of it.

I had almost no peers in the area: a small community of bungalows populated by old and middle-aged Russians, some of them with their children no older than age five. One dimwitted boy around my age would come for the weekends, and we played videogames together, but that was the extent of it. Only a few houses down, however, there were two girls, cousins, who were also spending the summer there, living with just the ancient grandmother of the eldest, who rarely if ever ventured outside of her bedroom, where she appeared to do nothing but watch TV.

I wasn't very attracted to the older cousin, who was one or two years my elder, and (in a small bit of irony) had herself had a long history of depression, and a few failed suicide attempts under her belt. From what I could tell, she didn't especially like me either. But the younger cousin, let's call her Y, certainly did catch my attention. She was quite attractive, physically well-developed, with large breasts on an athletic body, and—what was perhaps most important to my past self—she was exactly my age.

The three of us—Y, her older cousin, and I—began to hang out together almost every day. At some point during that time, Y started to like me, and I noticed. We would play games together in which I'd try my best to get a rise out of her: to startle her, or spray her with water, or seemingly accidentally touch her body. She responded to this very positively and even appeared to enjoy it.

In my interior life, I soon grew very excited at the prospect of winning Y over to become my girlfriend. She would be my first, and it would certainly give me something to brag to my friends about. Some of my friends had already had girlfriends, and some had already had sex. I was enormously eager to join that club, and to get ahead of those friends who had not yet had girlfriends or lost their virginity—something that I planned to hold over them as a grand superiority. This was, and had for a long time been, a major goal of mine.

One afternoon, I decided to take the next step, and put my arm around Y while the three of us sat on their couch watching TV—the ancient grandmother hidden safely away in her bedroom. Y didn't protest this action, and instead drew closer to me in response. My heart raced in my chest.

Several days after that, I finally gathered the courage to kiss her. She didn't protest this act either, and reciprocated the kiss eagerly. It was sealed. We spent the next couple weeks walking hand in hand, making out, and watching TV in each other's arms, mostly away from the older cousin. I enjoyed all this immensely; it was a new and extremely exciting time in my life.

Very notably, we did all of this without talking much. Whenever we did talk, it was largely idle and trivial conversation. We literally never, not once, explicitly discussed anything about our relationship. I remember one time wanting to tell her, explicitly, that I was her boyfriend, but then found myself too anxious to say it. Anything on the topic was only briefly mentioned or alluded to in the buffering presence of Y's cousin, who still hung out with us from time to time, but increasingly less often.

Y and I would meet one another at some point every day, and then decide to go for a walk in the forest, or watch television, or go to some other place where we'd invariably make out and cuddle, but without once speaking of any intention to do so or making any verbal reference to it during. It all appeared implicitly understood between us.

(In a similar vein, I also avoided looking at Y's face whenever I could: she had a large, Jewish nose that I didn't find especially pleasant to look at.)

Although the time we spent together only encompassed a portion of each day, I had no thoughts to spare for anything else. I completely neglected every book I intended to read, and spent most of my time looking forward to when I'd see Y again—all the time planning and contemplating what was the best way, place, and time to go about having sex with her. I felt that I'd already shied away from several good opportunities to do so (times when my hand was halfway down her panties, but I was lacking the nerve to go further), and finally steeled my courage to make a wholehearted attempt at it. It had already been nearly a month since we started seeing each other, and I thought that the time had to be now or never.

One night, while we were making out and cuddling together, she was laying on top of me on her bed, I decided to take things further, and made an attempt to unhook her bra and remove her shirt. This time, she quickly recoiled, and clearly rejected my advances. I calmly accepted that this simply wasn't the right time—and attached no special importance to it—since we continued to French kiss and cuddle the rest of the night as if nothing had happened. It was only when I kissed her goodbye that night, and her lips felt a little different, a little stiffer, a little less responsive, that I suspected that something might indeed be wrong. But then I decided that she was just flustered, and thought nothing further of it.

The next day, however, Y didn't answer my calls and, for the first day in two or three weeks, we didn't see each other. The same thing happened the next couple of days, and when I tried to go see her in person, she'd tell me through her doorway something to the effect of being busy, shut the door, and retreat back into her house. Finally, when I intercepted her in the road and implored her to discuss what was happening, she replied that she had no desire to talk to me and forcefully ignored me the rest of the time. This was especially effective because of the presence of her older cousin, who seemed to have formed an alliance with Y against me.

I was both puzzled and angered by this. I spent full days obsessing over it, forming different theories about what change might have occurred in Y that made her react to me in this way. My first guess was that it was caused by my trying to have sex with her that night. I also suspected that her older cousin might have convinced her I was despicable in some way. My best hypothesis was a combination of the two. I also thought Y might simply be on her period, which was making her act in an unexpected manner.

In any case, when my attempts to find out the cause and remedy the situation failed, I decided that trying to pursue this any further would be a pathetic and demeaning action on my part. The whole time our flimsy relationship lasted, I took pride in the notion that I didn't feel much of anything toward Y; and I'd often tell myself that I meant more to her than she did to me. I certainly enjoyed our time together, but it was mainly the process of making out and groping her that I enjoyed; Y was simply the person I had the opportunity to do it with. I also took pleasure in just the idea that I had a girlfriend. Her presence, I'd frequently tell myself, was what was important to me at the time, the girl herself wasn't. I felt that any great effort to win her back would be admitting the opposite, and decided that I could easily find another girl if I returned to the city.

So, finally acting on my pride and anger, I abandoned the situation entirely. I asked my parents to bring me back to the city, they obliged, and I never saw Y again.

A short while after returning home, I suddenly felt my life to be purposeless. I found myself oddly unable to derive pleasure from my favorite activities, and had no idea why this was happening to me. I'd hang out with my best friends, most of whom had already returned from camp, and go to the movies and play handball with them, all the while feeling it empty, pointless, and bereft of enjoyment. I yearned for the exciting process of cultivating and furthering a romantic relationship with the final goal of sex. Compared to that, anything I had the opportunity to do while at home seemed utterly meaningless to me.

I didn't find another girl, and looked back with reproach and self-criticism at each time I might have squandered my chance to have sex with Y—as well as the awkward, dishonest, or abrasive ways I sometimes behaved toward her. I often thought back with stinging reproach at the one night I tried to have sex with Y, and fretted over the fact that I could've gone about it a lot smarter. I thought about all the ways I could've repaired the problem, the things I could've said to Y or her cousin to clear matters up, or that it might have been only a matter of waiting out Y's period, and not leaving so impulsively and abruptly. All this was thoroughly infused with reproach emotion.

Every time I thought about my desires for sex and romance, which was almost always, my thoughts eventually came back to Y. And every time I thought about Y, I'd invariably feel a cascade of regret, sadness, and self-reproach, and then force all those thoughts out of my mind.

As the summer progressed, and most of my friends again left the city, I began having a very hard time simply leaving my house. I did force myself to do so every single day, and went to a nearby park to play handball until sundown, but each time required an enormous effort. Playing handball every day, sometimes all day, I became remarkably good at the game, but experienced almost no pleasure from it. I did have some fleeting minutes of enjoyment, when I was with friends, or during especially intense games at the park, when all my attention was absorbed in something external to me, but that enjoyment would fade almost instantly the second I became conscious of it, and saw that it was basically purposeless.

There were, however, a couple prospects of finding another girlfriend during this period—a girl I met at the park or saw in my neighborhood—about which I'd get extremely excited for several days at a time. But these never materialized into anything, and I'd sink once again into dejection and anhedonia.

What I experienced was, clearly, the typical picture of a mild depression. This lasted for about two months, during which time I periodically scoured the internet in an attempt to find news about what Y was doing and what made her become so harshly disposed toward me. Finally, after two months of searching, I came upon a short conversation between Y and her older cousin on an online forum I knew they both frequented, and also what their usernames were. It was a brief exchange, of no more than a few sentences, in which they clearly referred to me, and denounced me as a typical guy who only wanted sex.

With this, my depression was cured instantly, and with no residual side effects. I had received confirmation—a definite closure—that it was indeed due to my sexual advances that Y turned on me so abruptly. And that absolved me of all self-reproach. The opportunity to have sex and lose my virginity, which I thought I so foolishly squandered, had been a dead end the whole time. Y never intended to have sex with me, no matter what way I had gone about it. I thus achieved a genuine reevaluation of my loss: the reevaluation that there really was nothing to lose in the first place, and that I got everything out of the relationship that I possibly could have. This gave me a great joy, and I promptly returned to being my usual, witty, cheery self.

I have never experienced depression since.

This instant curing of my depression perfectly demonstrates the power of reevaluation. And the astounding thing is that its effect was purely psychological. Nothing about my situation actually changed. I still didn't have a girlfriend, and I was still a virgin. Only now, I saw this to be unavoidable, and that it wasn't my own fault.

It is these kinds of sudden reappraisals that psychologists haven't been able to pin down as the true cause of some people's spontaneous recoveries from depression. And that is what gives me such confidence in the efficacy of introspection to answer the questions academic psychology hasn't been able to.

I shall discuss some other reevaluations able to cure depression in the final part of this book.

Chapter 10

Secondary Symptoms

There are some additional symptoms and elements of depression that I haven't addressed yet. I will do so now. I don't think these symptoms are among the primary causes of depression, and consider them to be merely secondary, emergent properties of the condition. They are, however, often prominent in the behavior of depressed persons, and inspecting them further should prove highly instructive.

Manic Depression

The first issue I wish to address is the uncanny tendency for some depressed people's illness to assume a bipolar nature. It's true that some people's depression, about 10 to 20 percent of all cases, will later transform into manic depression, in which episodes of intense sadness, self-hate, and anhedonia (depression) typically alternate with episodes of intense excitement, elation, and self-esteem (mania). Although this might seem highly paradoxical, the reasons for it should become evident once we examine the psychological causes of mania.

When a person obtains something that he desires, the fulfillment of a wish, he experiences what we may call undifferentiated happiness. He smiles, his eyes light up, he feels an inner state of joy, warmth, and overall wellbeing. Then, depending on what he attributes this satisfaction to, his happiness will acquire a secondary dimension.

If he sees his wish-fulfillment as caused by another person—if it was, for instance, a gift from a friend—his happiness will become mixed with affection, love, and gratitude to that other person. If he sees his wish-fulfillment as the result of luck, chance, or fate, his happiness will become mixed with a feeling of awe, blessedness, and good fortune. And if he sees his wish-fulfillment as being caused by himself, by his own actions and efforts, his happiness will become modified by a feeling of self-esteem. Kay Redfield Jamison, the foremost expert on manic-depression, and a manic-depressive herself, has fittingly named this emotion of happiness augmented by self-esteem: "exuberance."

And that is, essentially, what mania is. It is the psychological state of a person experiencing an intense and prolonged period of happiness and/or excitement, augmented by self-esteem. That individual feels elated, confident; he feels that he's able to take on anything, overcome any challenge; the future looks bright to him; he senses his own importance. These are, of course, the natural effects of exuberance, but they also qualify a person for the diagnosis of mania—at least when experienced in excess. "Mania," according to Jamison, "is exuberance gone amok."

In fact, the highest peaks of human experience are those of mania. But it's frequently deemed pathological because it causes some people, in their elation, to engage in reckless, risk-taking behavior; to form harmful, delusional beliefs; and to commit selfish, antisocial actions. Some of the common pitfalls of mania include getting into a car accident due to reckless driving; catching a sexually transmitted disease from having unprotected sex with strangers; carelessly spending, giving away, or gambling away all of your money; jumping out of a window believing you can fly; thinking that God is talking to you; thinking that you are God; damaging relationships with friends and family due to callous behavior; or severing those relationships willfully from a desire for independence. In some cases, intense mania directly sets off a psychotic episode—as all overwhelming emotions are capable of doing. Anger is also commonly present in mania, in the role of a complementary emotion.

The psychological triggers of the mania emotions (exuberant happiness and exuberant excitement) are as follows. The exuberant version of happiness is caused by achieving a desire or overcoming a hardship. It comes from a person's appraisal that he is himself responsible for his success, for his triumphs.[64] Exuberant excitement has a similar cause. It's triggered by the person anticipating those future achievements he thinks will produce in him this type of happiness. (And anger, which is often mixed in with mania, is frequently set off by obstacles that interfere with achieving that happiness.) It is, in fact, doubtful whether happiness and excitement, whatever their cause, are not just two manifestations of the same emotional reaction. I think that is highly probable. Nevertheless, the two produce markedly different effects on the human mind.

Happiness, or at least its exuberant variety, contains two tiers of affect. The first occurs immediately after the person achieves his triumph—it is deliverance. A rampant feeling of elation explodes within the person. He wants to express it, to jump, to scream, to celebrate. He finds it hard to stay still. His thoughts race. He wants to be active. Sleep is an utterly unattractive prospect for him. This lasts for a while, sometimes minutes, sometimes hours, sometimes days, depending on the person and the size of the triumph; but it eventually fades and gives way to the second tier of exuberance. Here the person feels calm, content, at peace. He is perfectly able to stay in place; he is collected. It is a meditative-like state. Thoughts and ideas come freely and easily. The person feels at one with the world and at the same time a detached observer of it. Events that would otherwise evoke another emotion in him (anger, anxiety, and so on)

---

[64] That assessment is really identical to the one that evokes the reproach emotion: seeing oneself as the cause (or one of the causes) of an event. But in self-reproach it's an unpleasant, negative event, and in happiness blended with self-esteem it must be a positive, pleasant event.

no longer do. He feels passive, serene, and is deeply contemplative. Eventually this fades as well, and the person returns to his normal state.

The exuberant type of excitement has a similar initial effect. Here the person hasn't achieved a triumph, but is infatuated with the idea of a future one. He too feels an eager exhilaration brewing within him. He too has a hard time containing it and wants to jump, run, and celebrate. He finds it hard to stay still and his thoughts race. He feels capable, confident, and the future looks bright. Unlike happiness, however, this excitement is inseparably linked to the thoughts and ideas that evoke it. Once the exciting idea leaves the person's mind, the affect of excitement follows almost immediately behind it. There is little or no second tier, and the person reverts to his normal mental state as soon as the initial burst of excitement is over. This, nevertheless, can still qualify for a diagnosis of mania.

We can now see a close parallel between the emotions of happiness and excitement, augmented by self-esteem, and the emotion of sadness, augmented by self-reproach. The former are the result of victory and hope, while the latter is the result of defeat and the loss of hope. They are, after all, but the two outcomes of the same battle. A person's efforts at a goal can either end in victory or defeat; his hopes for the future can either be stoked or shattered. Returning now to the topic of depression, we can see why a depressed person's intense sadness can sometimes be replaced by an intense excitement or joy: mania.

The depressed person consumed with sadness after a loss, in our example the loss of a romantic relationship, will instinctively seek to regain what he lost. That is his battle. His depression remains precisely because he's unable to do so, unable to find a new romantic relationship. But his depression spans a long period of time. And in this time, there will likely be moments when he sees a chance of winning his battle: an opportunity. He meets a girl or gets a call from his ex-girlfriend. In my own case, I'd get extremely excited for days when I foresaw the prospect of finding another girl. And though this didn't quite reach the level of mania, I can certainly see how it could've, if those prospects had a much better chance of becoming real. In any case, for a depressed person, it's clearly appropriate for this type of excitement to be highly intense and all-consuming—since, for him, he sees a real chance to shed all his problems and obtain what he really wants, perhaps the only thing that he really wants.

Of course, these periods of excitement are bound to revert back to depression if the desired outcome doesn't transpire and he is once again disappointed.[65] But if the desired outcome *is* realized, and the person does get what he wants, his depression will likely be cured then and there (unless that desire was misdirected).

And this brings up another feature of depression I touched upon earlier in this book: the gap in some depressed people's anhedonia. This is a unique attitude the depressed person holds toward a particular topic—one to which he reacts peculiarly, perhaps even passionately, in contrast to the general anhedonic attitude he has toward everything else. I first mentioned my strong suspicion that this topic is usually closely linked to the cause of the person's depression. I later discussed how, in the depression caused by the loss of an immature romance, this topic tends to be anything related to finding a new one. We can see its broader implications here.

In cases of depression in general, this topic is one of regaining or replacing the loss of whatever brought on the depression. To this topic, we can expect the person to initially react with excitement,

---

[65] It is for this same basic reason that the normally manic person will likely, at some point, be hit with an episode of depression. If there is something at which he is constantly succeeding, and which provides him with such intense feelings of happiness, excitement, and self-esteem, on the occasion he fails at it (which is bound to happen at some point in time) he will be inclined to experience an equally strong feeling of sadness.

perhaps even mania.[66] It frequently happens, however, that after the person has been depressed for a long time, that excitement becomes inhibited by a different negative emotion, usually anxiety. (That is typically what occurs when the depressed person's attempts to regain what he lost are constantly disappointed and his manic expectations never pan out.)

It's in these peculiar attitudes, especially those that result in episodes of excitement or mania, that we have the greatest opportunity to determine the event that caused a person's depression. If we're fortunate enough to catch a depressed person during these manic episodes, or to coax him to reminisce upon such an occasion, it's bound to yield invaluable clues about his condition. We should look for what the person seeks in those instances. What does he want? What thoughts occupy his mind? Undoubtedly, that information would be of great therapeutic value.

Anger

The next issue I wish to address is the presence of anger in depression, especially the depression that stems from an immature breakup. There is, in fact, often an element of anger in depression—in the depressions produced by an immature breakup, it is anger directed at the ex-partner. This anger can manifest itself in at least three different ways.

The first way is as an undertone to the dominating emotion of self-reproach. Although the depressed person usually blames the breakup on himself—the direction exactly opposite of anger—the situation, in reality, isn't so strictly dichotomous. We may rightfully say that this person primarily casts blame on himself, but not that he does so exclusively. It may very well happen, and it may even be likely, that the person will *also* cast blame on his former partner—or

---

[66] While that person may, it is true, attempt to suppress this excitement in front of others, his attempts to suppress it will also, in all likelihood, be noticeably different from his usual anhedonic attitude.

at least some portion of it. After all, the event of a breakup (and any event for that matter) is not a one-dimensional thing: It is nuanced. And it is certainly possible, and quite understandable, if the person was to be angry at his ex-partner for the role that she played in the breakup, and reproachful at himself for the role that he played in it. (Also, just as by sheer virtue of time, the history of almost any relationship is bound to contain some past events for which the person reproaches himself, so is it bound to include some other events that evoke anger toward his ex-partner. The depressed person, whose sadness compels him to dwell on his relationship's past, may now recall those angering experiences, and thereby revive some of that previous anger.)

The second way anger can be present in depression is, as I mentioned earlier, as one of the two emotional poles the person vacillates between when he is uncertain of who he should blame for the breakup. (John Bowlby showed this to be a fairly common reaction in people maladaptively grieving the death of a loved one.)

A third position anger can occupy in depression is, instead of the usual self-reproach, the main blame emotion the person will feel in response to the breakup. But while the vengeful breakup doesn't normally lead to depression, it certainly can when, in some cases, the person actually blames himself *for* feeling angry, which triggers a strong self-reproach that makes him repress both his loss and his reaction to it. He essentially winds up in the same psychological boat as the person who blames himself for his loss in the first place, but with an additional factor that doubly complicates matters. (This is, by the way, a classic example of a depression that's caused by a repression that's caused by an internal conflict with the Freudian superego.)

How large a factor anger is in a person's depression can therefore vary—from a faint, general undertone to his thoughts and behavior; to an intrusive, occasional presence in his mental life; to one of the dominating psychological aspects of his clinical disorder. Acknowledging that, we should likewise recognize that anger can be a peripheral motivation for the depressed person's uncanny acts of public self-abasement, self-harm, and even suicide.

Self-Harm and Suicide

Two dangerous behaviors stand out most markedly in depression: They are self-harm and suicide. Both are utterly appalling to the lay-person and run totally contrary to the most basic human (and animal) instincts to protect one's body and moreover one's life. But while these two behaviors appear cut from the same cloth, the motivation for each is, in fact, entirely different.

While a depressed person's main motivation for suicide is typically the emotion of sadness, his or her main motivation behind self-harm is usually the reproach emotion. A depressed person is drawn to suicide as a way to end his perpetual suffering. His daily experience is thoroughly saturated with painful emotion—mostly sadness, but also reproach emotion, and sometimes anxiety. For months or years he's been unable to remedy these feelings, which refuse to subside and only become more tenacious. This person suffers through each day and expects only more of such pain from each successive one. To escape his painful present and his painful future, he seeks suicide as his only foreseeable path to relief. It is really a misdirected instinct to avoid pain—an instinct of self-preservation that nonetheless leads to self-destruction.

Self-harm is a different story. Here the person doesn't seek a total abolition of pain. Instead, he inflicts minor injuries on himself. This is most often accomplished by using a blade to cut the skin and underlying tissue (usually on the arms or legs), but bruising, burning, hair-pulling, and other odd methods are sometimes employed as well. The main culprit in this is the reproach emotion. It is, after all, an impulse of aggression, similar to anger, only directed at oneself. Just as anger motivates a person to inflict harm on whomever incurred that anger, the reproach emotion compels him to inflict harm on himself. Such a compulsion is peripheral, and normally the reproach emotion doesn't lead to physical self-injury.[67] But when it's experienced fiercely and for a prolonged period of time, which is exactly what happens in depression when the competing emotion of sadness makes the person dwell on reproachful memories instead of dismissing them outright, the person driven to express his reproach emotion may find his most easily accessible option in self-harm.

And such self-harm *does* provide a temporary relief to his reproach emotion. It causes the person to shift his focus from his reproachful memories to the self-inflicted injury, the physical pain of which becomes a temporary symbol, a stand-in, for his regretted past actions. All that this person accomplishes here is replacing an emotional pain with a physical one, but it's a gain nevertheless since that new pain is surely the lesser one.[68] The problem is that, unlike anger, the reproach emotion is not satiated by doing punitive harm to oneself. And as a result, the person must repeatedly inflict new flesh wounds (once the pain of the old ones fades) to obtain the temporary relief he seeks from his self-reproaches.

It also frequently happens that the act of self-harm actually becomes *pleasurable* to the person. Rather, the pain it naturally causes becomes mixed with pleasure. Injuring oneself, after all, provides a calming sensation; it releases endorphins. And when the person's body eventually becomes acclimated to the self-inflicted physical pain, and dulls its intensity, the pleasure it provides overtakes the

---

[67] It's normally limited to verbal self-abuse. Just as anger compels a person to insult another, the reproach emotion compels him to insult himself.

[68] This is partially because a person who continually experiences the same negative affect—be it physical pain, emotional pain, nausea, starvation, or cold—becomes over time less and less tolerant of it, and the same amount of that pain begins to have a much more debilitating, taxing effect on him (it becomes much less bearable). This is certainly the case with the depressed person who's constantly plagued with reproach emotion. But it's also true that, in most cases, completely physical pain is simply, by its nature, more benign than emotional pain, especially the toxic pain of self-reproach.

pain it produces and the act becomes effectively pleasurable.[69] It may even become addictive, and the person might come to crave the calming sensation he gets from self-harm the same way a smoker craves a cigarette.

But let's not forget the peripheral motivation of anger. Both suicide and self-harm can also be used as a proxy for getting revenge. Depressed persons may covet the idea of using their own misery, even their deaths, as a way of hurting and incurring the guilt of others. To those whose depression is the result of an ended relationship, it's usually their ex-partner that they wish to harm in this way.[70]

That's not to say that revenge is a main motivating force that leads depressed people to such self-destructive behavior. Many perfectly healthy people have similar impulses in the course of their lives, without ever coming close to acting on them.[71] But, as we know, it's in the nature of motivation to stack up: for there to be multiple different sources fueling a behavior. And to the depressed

---

[69] This statement that a person's body becomes less sensitive to pain that's repeatedly experienced may seem like a contradiction of the last footnote, in which I stated that pain, when continually experienced, becomes more and more *unbearable* over time. Both statements, however, are true.

Most painful affects, especially when they occur contrary to the person's volition, become psychologically less bearable. The person becomes more conscious attuned to the pain, more sensitive, more aware of it. He pays more attention to it, and thus feels it more intensely. The pain occupies a more central position in his mind.

But it's also true that a person's *body* becomes less sensitive to certain kinds of physical pain when they're experienced often. People who frequently endure medical injections, extreme cold, extreme heat, electric shocks, physical impact from punches or kicks, or—for that matter—self-inflicted cuts, will grow much less sensitive to them over time.

[70] This, clearly, only pertains to cases in which that former partner is still in the depressed person's vicinity, when she is still bound to know about, and better yet care about, his fate.

[71] Most commonly this idea of harming or killing oneself in order to spite others is directed at one's parents, who have countless opportunities to incur their child's anger precisely because they care for his fate, and thus also stand to be damaged the most by his self-destructive actions.

person who already seriously entertains the idea of suicide, the peripheral motive of anger may very well give him the final push.

Public self-denigration, announcements of self-abasement, and declarations of one's own misery to friends and relatives (a very pronounced behavior in many depressed persons) can have this same motive as well. I will discuss that next.

Public Self-Denigration

I already described the self-hating, self-denigrating, self-castigating perspective that most depressed people hold, and that—in the majority of cases—they freely declare to the people around them. They openly regard themselves as worthless, vile, sinful, and so forth; an attitude completely opposite to the self-esteem seeking mentality of the average person.[72]

I observed that this attitude was characteristic of the reproach emotion, since only it was capable of having that effect on the human mind. And yet, this brings up another problem—because, while the self-denigration the depressed person expresses is certainly the product of the reproach emotion, the fact that he verbally announces it to others runs completely contrary to the reproach emotion. Normally, a person experiencing self-reproach will be extremely averse to disclosing his reproachful actions to others—he'll typically try to hide them and avoid the topic. Instead, the depressed person freely gives vent to his feelings of shame and self-hatred. Why?

We'll find the answer to this when we examine in closer detail the actual behavior of the depressed person. It is, after all, markedly different from the normal expression of self-reproach in more than one facet.

---

[72] These announcements most commonly occur in the later stages of a depression, when the person's friends and family are already fully aware of his condition, and he no longer needs to hide his misery from them.

First off, it is clear the depressed person truly believes those negative opinions of himself he expresses. He really does think that he's worthless, wretched, unlovable. The reproach emotion alone doesn't have this effect: It's usually limited to a particular action, a specific memory, and disappears once that memory exits the person's mind. It doesn't, under normal circumstances, so thoroughly usurp the person's self-image.

We can, however, see why this happens to a depressed person. After all, his reproach emotion is inseparably coupled with sadness. While a regular person seldom thinks of his past reproaches (in fact, he tries precisely not to think about them), the depressed person is, on the contrary, forced to dwell on them by a powerful emotion of sadness. As a consequence, his reproachful memories play a much greater role in his mental life, and he thus draws those negative conclusions from them as to the nature of his own character. But why does he, instead of concealing it, express his self-reproach to other people?

We may attribute this to the common human affinity for telling the truth over lying, since recalling the truth requires less mental effort than forming a lie. The depressed person thinks his own negative opinions of himself are true, and so he expresses them. But this only partly accounts for the facts. It can certainly be an active motivation when he's asked about himself by his friends and relatives; but most of the time, the depressed person announces these things unprovoked. It also doesn't appear that he's doing this to get those feelings off of his chest, so to speak. He shows no signs of relief from doing so, and continues to make the same announcements again and again to the same people.

What, then, drives the depressed person to brazenly announce the self-reproaches most others try hard to conceal? He certainly wishes most desperately to avoid any additional anguish (by way of a burning embarrassment) by also exposing his deepest, most regretted actions to the scrutiny of others. The answer is simple: He doesn't really expose them.

When we examine the depressed person's behavior more closely, we notice the self-denigrating announcements he makes to other people don't reference any specific acts or occurrences. They're always extreme generalities. "I'm worthless." "I'm incapable of love." "I can never do anything right." "I don't deserve to be happy." And so on and so forth.

But what happens if somebody challenges these assertions and asks him: Why? Almost invariably, the depressed person will fail to give a real explanation. He'll never disclose the specific reproachful actions from which he drew his conclusions. He'll likely respond with only more generalities, and try to assure the questioner that his self-denigrating assertions are right, that he knows himself well and it's just his inherent nature, and so on and so forth. Under normal conditions, it's close to impossible to get any specific details out of him.

As it turns out, the depressed person hides and avoids discussing his *actual* reproachful memories the same way any other person does—and likely a lot more fervently, since his are that much more painful. His public lamentations expound, instead, on the wider conclusions he formed about himself, and it's not these the reproach emotion renders taboo. *That* is the reason he feels no embarrassment from expressing his self-castigation in front of others: He doesn't actually reveal anything of an intimate nature. And that's also why he fails at getting those memories off his chest: If he did, his friend's and relative's understanding and acceptance of them would likely help him reach a reevaluation.

As for what motivations do drive the depressed person to give vent to his dismal self-image, we can now recognize them clearly. I already mentioned revenge as a possible motivation; but his main motive is clearly a want of sympathy.

The depressed person seeks sympathy from others through his behavior. He derives a slight instinctual pleasure, as most of us are prone to do, from having others share in his misery. In all of his vocal laments and self-criticisms, he's really just complaining to people, plainly fishing for whatever sympathy he can get—perhaps the one tiny pleasure, or relief from pain, he still has access to. And even when he seeks to satisfy a peripheral motivation of anger, he does so through sympathy as well—hoping to get a minor revenge on the person his anger's directed at by having that sympathy turn into guilt.

And so, there we have the solution to the depressed person's public lamentations. In expressing only his overall judgments and generalities, he still protects the core memories they sprang from in accordance with the reproach emotion. He thus uses them as a way to draw on the sympathy of others, without disclosing any of the actual details of his reproachful past actions.

We shouldn't, however, assume a depressed person does this deliberately—that is, consciously. In most cases, the depressed person himself doesn't realize what lies behind his dismal self-assessment, the reproachful memories, and only gives vent to the conclusions he draws from them as he himself sees them.[73] At the same time, this person subconsciously defends against calling up, and even more so discussing, any reproachful actions the same way everyone else tends to. His need for sympathy is also, in most cases, unconscious. We would be wise, therefore, *not* to consider this depressive behavior deceitful, and should assume, as a default, that the person is innocent of any duplicity.

Loss of Self-Esteem

On the one hand, the depressed person hates, blames, and vilifies himself—what we may call negative self-esteem. On the other hand, he thinks he has lost all abilities, virtues, and possibilities for the future—what we may consider a lack of positive self-esteem. The former, we know, is caused by the reproach emotion—by blaming

---

[73] It's actually a natural human tendency, in regular life and even in purely academic endeavors, for people to forget the original evidence and chain of logic behind a conclusion, and only remember the conclusion itself.

himself for his various failures. The latter, however, is much more an accurate appraisal of reality—based on the person's actual observations of his behavior, abilities, and mentality, while in the middle of a depressive episode.

Depression truly does rob a person of his abilities and motivation, often rendering him unable to even get out of bed. Observing this, the depressed person adjusts his self-concept (and his projection of the future) accordingly, and his positive self-esteem plummets. He thus concludes he is worthless, hopeless, and powerless.

The manic person does the same thing, but in exactly the opposite direction. Mania makes a person ultra-productive, creative, and motivated—it practically bestows him with superpowers. Observing this, he adjusts his self-concept (and his view of the future) accordingly, and his positive self-esteem surges. He concludes he is flawless, unstoppable, and has limitless potential.

The problem is, the human mind can't anticipate future emotional states. People unconsciously project the way they are feeling *now* on every scenario in the future. Thus, the manic person thinks he'll be manic always, constructs his self-concept on that assumption, and plans his whole life on that basis. The depressed person thinks his depression is permanent, constructs his self-concept on that premise, and decides he might as well end his life, since the future contains nothing else for him.

Both are mistaken to the extent that these mental states aren't permanent—and for virtually all individuals, neither mania or depression lasts forever. The manic person, therefore, overestimates his abilities and his forecasts of the future, and typically ends up disappointed when his mania disappears and he loses its quickening influence (a reversal that can, in itself, precipitate a depression). The depressed person, too, incorrectly appraises himself and his future, and when his depression eventually remits, he'll typically realize that he was selling himself short.

The key is to rationally understand that these states are only temporary, and neither foreclose on one's future and self-esteem, or inflate them to unrealistic levels of grandiosity, knowing that these states are bound to pass—even though, at the present moment, one's unconscious mind can provide no indication of this.

Chapter 11

When Depression Becomes Recurrent

As Richard O'Connor points out, for many individuals, "depression is a chronic disease that waxes and wanes over a lifetime." This is true. Each Major Depressive Episode, whatever else it may do, alters a person's brain structure, making it more reactive to stress, and increases the likelihood of another Major Depressive Episode.

With every Major Depressive Episode a person has, it takes a smaller and smaller provoking event to set off the next one. It might, therefore, take a major tragedy to precipitate a person's first episode of depression; a minor tragedy to set off his second one; a slight disappointment to set off his third; and practically nothing to set off his fourth, fifth, sixth, and so on.

Hence, a person who's had one Major Depressive Episode, has—on average—a 50 percent chance of having another one. A person who's had two Major Depressive Episodes, has a 70 percent chance of having a third. A person who's had three Major Depressive Episodes, has a 90 percent chance of having a fourth. And a person who's had four or more Major Depressive Episodes, is almost 100 percent guaranteed to have even more.

In this way, major depression often becomes a chronic, recurring condition—in which the person cycles between episodes of depression and periods of remission over the course of his life. From this, Richard O'Connor concludes that once "some stress pushes us over into our first real depression," there's usually no going back. Most people, then, simply "have" depression—the same way one can have herpes. Even after the manifest illness has passed, and the person's entirely free of symptoms, the disease is still there inside of him, ready to flare up again in response to some stressor.

Richard O'Connor calls these people "depressives," which I think is a highly apt term. Not only are they highly vulnerable to depression, and frequently experience Major Depressive Episodes, but even during their periods of remission they're typically stuck with "a low-grade dysthymia always there in the background that wasn't there before." These people, indeed, retain many depressive character traits—symptoms, beliefs, thought patterns, defenses, and insecurities—even while not clinically depressed: what may rightly be called a *depressive personality*. (This is something I observed extensively, first-hand, with my present girlfriend.)

The lives of most depressives therefore consist of a somewhat neurotic, maladjusted, general unhappiness when they're relatively well, peppered now and again with acute episodes of major depression. And with every successive episode, the next episodes tend to be shorter, closer together, and more intense. (This is why I consider the new DSM-5 category of "Persistent Depressive Disorder" both valid and valuable.) The best predictor of whether a person's depression will become recurrent is the duration of his first episode.[74]

---

[74] Although the literature doesn't address this, this process must occur differently in people with different genetic makeups. The New Zealand longitudinal study, which examined the effects of two versions of a serotonin-transporter gene on people's chance of developing depression, showed that exposure to a large stressor only slightly increased the risk of depression in persons with one genotype, yet greatly increased the risk in those with a different genotype (see page 24). And that's only one gene out of the hundreds likely involved in depression. It's certainly clear that, simply due to their DNA, some people will get depressed much more easily than others. Some may, therefore, require more Major Depressive Episodes, and of a longer duration, to become "depressives." Others may retain more or less the same chance of developing depression, however many episodes they've

Rumination and the Positive Feedback Loop

But it isn't just stress reactivity that makes chronic depressives so readily susceptible to Major Depressive Episodes. That's only half the story. The second half is a positive feedback loop established by habit in the chronic depressive's mind: the so-called "downward spiral" of depression, along which lies a variable sequence of the depressive's thoughts, feelings, reactions, and behavior.

A positive feedback loop is a runaway process taking place in a system that receives an input, amplifies it, and spits out that amplified form as its output. If that amplified output then feeds into the system again, without first being dampened to less than or equal to its initial level, and this process is permitted to loop continuously, the original input will be amplified to its physical limit, until it destroys the system entirely, or something else interferes to disrupt the process. This is how putting a microphone to its own speaker often burns out the speaker; how a small vibration, building on itself, collapses a bridge; and how purified uranium, when it reaches critical mass, produces a nuclear explosion. This is also what happens in

---

had previously. And others might be immune to depression entirely, no matter what horrible things happen to them.

The statistic that people who've had four or more Major Depressive Episodes have nearly a hundred percent chance of having another does not contradict these possibilities. People whose likelihood of developing depression remains constant (or increases only slightly) with each Major Depressive Episode may have had four or more episodes merely by chance: resulting from four depression-worthy catastrophes in their lives. Although their chance of having another episode might be quite small, their initial chance of having four episodes is likewise extremely small, making the few of them that did an insignificant blip in the data. This is the classic logical fallacy—so often committed in modern psychology—of assuming that group statistics apply to all individuals, since there may exist some individuals that do not conform to the group trend, yet are lost in the data as a tiny minority. Whether there are depression-resistant individuals like this, however, is only a matter of conjecture. And since there isn't good information about this, I am withholding my judgment.

depression; because, as we saw earlier, the symptoms of depression also cause and intensify depression.

Psychologists have adopted the term "rumination" to refer to this downward spiral, which captures its essence well. It consists of brooding upon some unpleasant experience, emotion, or cognition; then self-critically analyzing what it means about oneself, the world, and one's future; then having even more painful thoughts, feelings, and experiences as a result of that unsparing analysis; then dwelling, worrying, and obsessing over what that rapidly sinking mood implies about one's self-worth, one's place in the world, and one's possibilities for happiness; then feeling even worse as a result of that questioning; then questioning the repercussions of that even further; and then finally, at the end, finding that one has imperceptibly descended into a full-blown clinical depression.

A person might, for example, visit a new auto shop, where the mechanic is rude to him and overcharges him for an oil change. On the drive home, feeling angry, ashamed, and humiliated, he thinks: "The mechanic sees me as a nobody." He recalls similar instances in the recent and distant past where people disregarded, snubbed, or took advantage of him. "Nobody takes me seriously. No one respects me. Even my so-called friends secretly hate me." He imagines his friends laughing and making fun of him if they learned of his oil change rip-off. "I didn't even stand up for myself. I'm simply incapable of asserting myself. I'm such a wimp." He begins to feel anxious, the worry spreading to other elements of his life. "That's probably why I didn't get that promotion at work. That's probably why I'll never get one. They might even fire me soon. And since I can't even assert myself, I'll never be able to find another job." He returns home and plops on his couch feeling discouraged, exhausted, and sad. He had other chores he wanted to do that day, but now has no energy to do them. "I can't even manage the simplest tasks. I'm so lazy. No woman will ever want to date me again. Girls only like strong, confident, successful men, and not lazy, pathetic, prospectless wimps like me." He might go to sleep that day, but wake up in an equally lousy, disheartened, beaten down mood the next morning.

"Why am I like this? I'm never going to be happy. Why can't I be just like other, normal people? I'm going to die broke, miserable, and alone. I might as well kill myself." And so on and so forth.

This is how a chronic depressive's later depressive episodes can be triggered by something as insignificant as a small disappointment, an offhand comment, a random snub—or even something he read, or a song he heard, or a memory evoked by association. That essentially anything is able to trigger these later episodes, therefore, means that their proximal cause is much less the events that precipitate them, and almost entirely the positive feedback mechanism that's been assembled in the depressive's mind. And that is exactly the mark the initial few Major Depressive Episodes leave on a person: they lay down the mental machinery of his positive feedback loop, which leads him down the downward spiral of rumination that amplifies minor events into major depressions.

These previous episodes really do three things, each of which reinforces a different part of the feedback loop. Imagine a regular handheld microphone with its cable plugged in to a large loudspeaker. First, a Major Depressive Episode is a highly stressful experience, which changes the biochemistry of a person's brain, and makes him a lot more reactive to future stressors. This corresponds to turning the volume up on the loudspeaker, so that all input received by the microphone is amplified to a higher intensity. Second, a Major Depressive Episode strengthens the associative connections between negative mood, self-critical thoughts, depressive beliefs, defensive reactions, feelings of worthlessness, forecasts of hopelessness, and all other components of the positive feedback loop, so that each one—when activated—more rapidly, strongly, and automatically triggers the others. (This happens because the more often certain thoughts, feelings, reactions, and so on are experienced together, the more the physical, neurological circuitry that links them becomes reinforced—essentially ingraining such thinking patterns into the brain as mental habits.) This corresponds to bringing the microphone physically closer to the loudspeaker, so that the sound has a smaller distance to travel and less dampening can occur before the speaker's output feeds into the microphone again. And third, the person's initial one or two Major Depressive Episodes actually *originate* the various mental elements that comprise the machinery of his positive feedback loop. This corresponds to obtaining and assembling the physical hardware of microphone, cable, speaker, and so on, which makes the positive feedback loop they can create possible.

Aaron Beck, the founder of Cognitive Behavioral Therapy for depression, calls this machinery a cognitive "constellation" of "interrelated negative attitudes," including false, oversimplified, negative beliefs about oneself, the world, and the future; a primitive tendency toward self-blame; and dreary expectations of failure for all of one's hopes and aspirations. Richard O'Connor calls the different parts of this positive feedback loop the "skills of depression," among which he also includes maladaptive behaviors, defense mechanisms, and modes of relating to other people that only promote and perpetuate depression. With each successive Major Depressive Episode, more and more parts of this cognitive constellation, or skills of depression, fall into place—until, after several episodes, the positive feedback loop is perfected.

And it isn't just Major Depressive Episodes that lay down these "skills," these separate pieces of—to use Aaron Beck's term—the "predepressive constellation." Traumatic events that *don't* lead to depression, like Adverse Childhood Experiences, also leave behind various maladaptive beliefs, defenses, behaviors, and insecurities, which can form part of the positive feedback loop, and make people more vulnerable to depression later in life. And so, for that matter, can regular learning. Children can, for instance, learn false depressive beliefs about themselves, the world, and other people directly from their parents. They can also model ineffective, self-defeating behaviors on those of their parents. And their parents may fail to provide them with the positive experiences required for healthy psychological growth—including the development of a stable identity and self-esteem. All of this happens extremely often, and is one major reason why children of depressed mothers go on to have such high rates of depression.

And it isn't only depression these "skills" predispose people to. They are, after all, distinct elements of a general neuroticism: maladaptive ways of relating to the world, to other people, and to one's own mind, which causes the person unnecessary mental distress. This general neuroticism, or poor psychological health, is the soil in which acute psychological illnesses like to take root, and does often diversify into these specific mental disorders. That's a big reason why depression is so often comorbid with other psychological illnesses— including Post Traumatic Stress Disorder, Obsessive-Compulsive Disorder, and all kinds of anxiety disorders.

Depression's Lasting Influence on My Life

In my case, my single episode of depression passed off completely. After it, I felt exactly the same as I did before, with no residual symptoms, and certainly no "low-grade dysthymia" floating around in the background. I seemed to have made a total recovery; and only much later did I notice the lasting effects this experience had on my life.

It was, for one thing, an unequivocal defeat in my pursuit of the opposite sex. And as all such defeats are liable to do, it markedly lowered my self-esteem, especially in that area. It made me feel, on the whole, less desirable to women, and certainly lowered my confidence in my ability to attract them. Furthermore, in being a defeat with such painful emotional repercussions, it sensitized me to similar failures and defeats in the future. It left me with a rather extreme and involuntary fear of rejection, a powerful *rejection sensitivity*, which placed me in the precarious position of feverishly craving romance with women, and at the same time morbidly fearing getting rejected by them. On top of all that, it instilled me with the pernicious belief, drawn solely from this single experience, that girls were generally hostile to sex: that they didn't like it and didn't want it (except under exceedingly favorable circumstances). Before that, I actually held the exact opposite belief: that girls wanted sex as much as men did; but now, my assumptions swung to the other extreme. This conclusion, despite all the evidence I could muster against it, was too emotionally compelling—on a purely unconscious, experiential level—for me to disbelieve. And from that point forward, I viewed my sexual desires for women not as a normal, mutually beneficial interest, but as a lascivious, predatory obsession—since the targets of these desires, the girls that I lusted after, would be repelled and horrified if they learned about them.[75]

The combined effect of all this was that I ended up pursuing girls, romance, and the goal of losing my virginity—which was, all throughout high school, the most important thing in my life—in a skulking, shame-filled, surreptitious way. I felt a compulsive need to deny, lie about, and conceal all sexual desires from the girls I liked—falsely pretending to be cold, aloof, and indifferent even while interacting with them—because, in my mind, they'd be appalled to discover what I was really thinking, which would lead to almost certain rejection if I asked them out on a date. And, if I ever did ask them out on a date, I felt totally paralyzed to do so openly and directly, which would expose me to outright, unmitigated rejection. I could only do so if I made it seem unintentional: perhaps "accidentally" running into the girl after school, and proposing—as if on a whim—that we go somewhere together; or maybe offhandedly broaching the topic in casual conversation, entirely nonchalantly, as if I just had the idea for the very first time. That way, even if I was refused, it would just be a meaningless event, and not a humiliating rejection, since—at least on the face of it—it wasn't something I was heavily invested in, but merely a whim I had on the spur of the moment. All of this was, of course, totally self-defeating; and I spent my final three years of high school a frustrated, neurotic, sex-obsessed virgin.

Although that personal example may be unimpressive, I think it still illustrates my key point: Despite fully recovering from my brief episode of depression, it nonetheless had a lasting, deleterious effect—making me more risk-avoidant in my sexual pursuits, less able

---

[75] This is a perfect example of how an evaluation drawn from an emotionally significant experience unconsciously and irresistibly transposes itself upon similar situations in the future.

to cope with future defeats and losses, and less competent in navigating life in general. It probably made me more vulnerable to more Major Depressive Episodes, as well as to other psychological disorders. (If several years later, I didn't injure my spine, which led me to a state of self-actualization, in which I confronted and resolved all my psychological problems, the residues of this period included, I think it is highly likely I would've become depressed again, and maybe again and again.)[76] In sum, it takes a lot more than to fully recover from the symptoms of a Major Depressive Episode to come to terms with and master the experience that caused it (or the experience of the episode itself).

---

[76] That experience, and the psychology of self-actualization, is the topic of my next book: *Self-Actualizing People in History*.

Chapter 12

The Different Types of Depression and What Cures Them

A lot has been written, in recent years, about chronic depression. Books like Richard O'Connor's *Undoing Depression*, Andrew Solomon's *The Noonday Demon*, and Mark Williams' *The Mindful Way Through Depression* describe the condition beautifully, dissect its causes brilliantly, and offer intelligent, tested, and genuinely effective remedies.

Richard O'Connor conceives the task of recovering from chronic depression as a matter of "replacing" the maladaptive, self-defeating, mutually-reinforcing "skills of depression" with new, healthy, effective skills of "thinking, feeling, and doing:" a process that he compares to unraveling "a big, intertwined ball of string," and which takes years upon years of persistent effort. Andrew Solomon likewise states, extremely astutely, that the best long-term remedy for depression is improving one's general psychological health in "between bouts of [major] depression." This includes, among other things, acquiring self-knowledge and developing new areas of competence. The most recent arrival on the scene of depression therapy, Mindfulness-Based Cognitive Therapy, delivers on that goal of self-knowledge in a big way. It teaches its patients "mindfulness meditation," a meditative practice for non-judgmentally observing one's own mental processes, including the mental process of rumination that sets off the downward spiral of depression. It also educates the person about the nature of the emotions and thought patterns he's observing, and thereby allows him to get an objective, detached perspective on them. The realization that "I am not my thoughts," which enables the person to *disidentify* with his depressive thought processes, and recognize that they are just "appearances in consciousness," and not the unvarnished truth about oneself, the world, and the future, is an enormous breakthrough for many depressed patients.

During periods of recovery, a chronic depressive's worldview—of himself, world, and future—typically reverts to more or less that of an average person. The difference is, as Richard O'Connor writes, that the depressive severely "lack[s] confidence in [his] own judgment." He's dreadfully unsure of his somewhat recovered sense of self-worth, his more benevolent view of reality, and his more optimistic belief in the future. And when a sad mood eventually rolls around, and sets off his habitual depressive beliefs—that he's worthless, his future is hopeless, and he is helpless in the face of reality—it's those that he now thinks are true. Mindfulness-Based Cognitive Therapy teaches him to distinguish his accurate, objective perceptions of reality from his temporary, emotionally compelling illusions—leaving him with a rather stable bedrock of truth that doesn't change with his fluctuating mood. It also enables the person to notice when he's beginning to ruminate, to identify that depressive reaction for what it is, and to break off that process at an early stage—interrupting the positive feedback loop before it can spiral down into depression.[77]

---

[77] In the mid-twentieth century, the behaviorist school of psychology supplanted the Freudian, declaring that all Freud's ideas were unscientific, and undertook to rebuild the science of psychology from a blank slate. This so-called "behaviorist revolution" succeeded, creating the modern, experimental psychology that still reigns today. And ever since then, psychologists have been furtively trying to sneak Freud's valuable, though officially heretical, concepts back into the fold of respectable psychology, but under

Mindfulness-Based Cognitive Therapy has proven impressively effective for treating recurrent depression. The eight-week mindfulness program laid out in *The Mindful Way Through Depression* has been shown—in multiple studies—to reduce the rate of relapse in the twelve-months following the treatment from 60 percent to 33 percent in patients with three previous episodes, and from 100 percent to 38 percent in those with at least four previous episodes. It hasn't, however, shown any effectiveness in patients with just two previous episodes; or those in the middle of a depressive episode; or for preventing an episode in the wake of a serious real-life stressor.

We know, thanks primarily to the mindfulness psychologists, that a recurrent episode of depression is usually caused by a runaway process of rumination that can be triggered by the most trivial event. This typically happens to people with multiple previous episodes of depression, who are high in neuroticism even during their periods of

---

a different guise. Mindfulness is one of these concepts, an extremely successful rebranding of what Freud would have called introspection; though it's also much more than that. It's not merely a new word for introspection, it's also a very specific—meditation centered—technique for introspection (and a very different technique from the one Freud used). Its basic effects, however, are essentially the same.

Mindfulness, state its advocates, is the cure to "experiential avoidance"—a person's attempts to avoid his thoughts, feelings, memories, and bodily sensations—which is another rebranding of a classic Freudian term: repression. By bringing a non-judgmental awareness to the experiences you are avoiding, they claim, you will see that you have nothing to fear from them, and be relieved of a great psychological burden. By making whatever you are repressing conscious, says Freud, you can replace the involuntary symptoms the repression was generating with logical understanding, and cease having to exert mental effort staving it off every time that it threatens to enter your thoughts.

Here I was proclaiming that introspective psychology's dead, right as the new mindfulness psychologists had managed to smuggle it in again through the back door. It is, of course, only a start toward a full science that includes introspection as a valid method. But seeing how quickly the mindfulness school gained academic acceptance, there might be some hope for mainstream psychology after all.

remission, and who usually have a history of some sort of childhood trauma.

The very first episode of depression, however, can occur to practically anybody, at any time, regardless of their age, their childhood experience, or even their psychological health. (The great Russian writer Aleksandr Solzhenitsyn, for example, had reached a state of full self-actualization—the highest level of psychological health available to a human being—when he was struck with his first, and only, Major Depressive Episode, set off when the KGB found and confiscated his secret manuscripts, which almost certainly boded his imminent arrest and the total destruction of his life's work.)

Practically nothing has been written in recent decades about this first episode of depression (which is, typically, a more or less understandable reaction to a serious internal or external event), and almost everything written in the decades before that has failed to give an adequate explanation of it. That is, of course, what the bulk of this book was about. And I now wish to end it by elaborating on its most crucial conclusions, and then briefly discussing the implications that those conclusions have for therapy.

When Depression is an Appropriate Reaction

While the depressive rumination that spirals down into a full-blown clinical depression is always an irrational, pathological response; a person's first, and even his second episode of major depression can be a fully appropriate—although likely ineffective—response to a real situation he finds himself in. It is, after all, an unavoidable consequence of three coexisting (and totally indispensable) human capacities: (1) to experience sadness in response to a loss, (2) to hold a hierarchy of values, and (3) to pass moral judgement.

The emotion of sadness is an instinctual reaction to the loss of something one values. If it isn't the loss of one's highest value, it will only result in a regular sadness—but no anhedonia. But a person ranks everything he values—by order of importance—in a hierarchy of values. This lets him set his priorities and make decisions in the face of alternatives, by implicitly informing him—usually by means of emotions—how important a certain goal is in comparison to others. If a person thus loses his highest value—something he thinks is supremely important or indispensable to him—and has no tangible hopes of getting it back, then it most likely will produce anhedonia, because nothing else matters in comparison. Morality, the final piece of the puzzle, is the instrument by which a person identifies the things, people, and actions beneficial to achieving his values—and the ones that are damaging. He judges the first to be moral, or *good*, and sets out to extoll and cultivate them; and judges the second to be immoral, or *evil*, and sets out to condemn and destroy them. If he, therefore, identifies his own self as the cause of losing his highest value, his moral judgment will label himself evil, and he'll essentially set out to destroy himself (often literally).

Morality is an enormously powerful force, at times for reverence and creation, at times for aggression and destruction. When a person blames himself for the loss of his top value, he labels his role in it a major sin, and turns his morality against himself. As one of the depressed soldiers in Aaron Beck's study—who inadvertently killed a friend by mistaking him for an enemy fighter—described his resultant depression and urge for self-punishment: "I am my own judge, jury and executioner." Sigmund Freud was perceptive as always when he proclaimed that depression was aggression turned inward.

Does it not make intuitive sense, then, that the person who ruined his life by his own actions would be depressed? Like the soldier who shot his best friend through the head and must now go to jail for it? Or the man who was texting his childhood sweetheart—the love of his life—while she was driving, "a bad habit we had," which then led to her fatal car crash? Does it not make perfect sense for this person to feel that his life's empty, meaningless, to be unable to draw pleasure from anything, and also to hate and want to kill himself? Imagine yourself in that same situation. How would you feel?

This isn't to say that one's first major depression is always, or even more than occasionally, a legitimate result of one's own tragic wrongdoing. It also depends, in large part, on how the person interprets the whole situation. If the person holds an irrational morality, he may illogically blame himself for a tragedy that wasn't his own fault. And if he holds an irrational hierarchy of values, he might consider a minor loss an insurmountable disaster. In that case, one's first major depression can certainly be irrational (like all other manifestations of human emotion)—and, in the vast majority of cases, it patently is.

The Three Types of Loss

Since the duration of one's first episode of major depression has such a large impact on whether the condition becomes chronic, it is especially important to provide quick and effective treatment for it. Knowing what we now know about the causes and psychology behind a first Major Depressive Episode, we can now form a pretty good idea of how this treatment should work and what it should strive to accomplish.

A first Major Depressive Episode, we know, nucleates around a large loss. And this loss can be of some thing in the past, the present, or the future.

A loss in the past is a loss that exists mainly in memory: one that no longer physically impacts one's day-to-day life. It can, for example, be the loss of a romantic relationship, which leaves the person about the same as he was before it (as happened in my case). Or it can be the death of a mother or father for an independent adult (as Freud had in mind when he wrote about "mourning" in *Mourning and Melancholia*).

A loss in the future is always the loss of a prospect: the loss of a plan, expectation, or hope that some beneficial thing will, in fact, happen. (This type of loss caused the depressions of Tolstoy, Ayn Rand, and John Stuart Mill.)[78]

---

[78] See footnote 58, page 97-98.

Finally, a loss in the present (if we may label it that) is a loss that continues to have an extensive, detrimental impact on the physical conditions of one's everyday life. This can be the loss of a job, which leaves one broke, homeless, or unable to feed one's children. It can be the loss of one's freedom, which leaves one spending his day-to-day life in prison. Or it can be the death of a parent in early childhood, which leaves the kid to grow up without a main caregiver, breadwinner, or role model. (Aleksandr Solzhenitsyn's depression was caused by this type of loss, when the KGB found and confiscated his secret manuscripts, which he thought would result in his imminent arrest.)

Every loss in the present, of course, also contains a memory of the event that caused it, as well as dashed hopes of a different and much better future. It will be useful, therefore, to talk about three dimensions of loss, and not just the three different types of losses. From this perspective, a loss in the past and a loss in the future are, in effect, special cases of loss that contain only one dimension. Still, these three separate types are very distinct psychologically, and the treatment of each should likewise be totally different. That is what I'll discuss next.

A Loss in the Past

A loss in the past produces a typical grieving response: The person feels an intense sadness from his awareness of the loss, and his attention is drawn to thoughts and memories of the lost relationship, person, or object. This grief is a natural coping mechanism, perhaps initially aimed at regaining or replacing the thing that was lost, but if that fails or is recognized as impossible, one that serves the adaptive function of understanding, coming to terms with, and adjusting to the new reality.

On its own, this is a perfectly healthy emotional reaction. It's telling, however, that it also can satisfy enough diagnostic criteria in the DSM to qualify for a Major Depressive Episode. At minimum, this healthy grief can produce: (1) a sad or depressed mood, (2) significant increase or decrease in appetite, (3) insomnia or hypersomnia, (4) fatigue or loss of energy, and (5) diminished ability to think or concentrate for most of the day, nearly every day, over a period of two weeks. This has been a lasting criticism of the DSM: that its reliance on a checklist of visible symptoms made normal grief "indistinguishable from depression." The DSM addresses this issue, however, by including a loophole known as "the bereavement exclusion." It states that a person may sometimes exhibit this classic (minimum) symptomology of major depression as "a normal reaction to the death of a loved one" and other "significant loss[es]," including "financial ruin, losses from a natural disaster, [or] a serious medical illness or disability"—exempting those afflicted with regular grief from being diagnosed with a mental illness.

This healthy reaction only turns pathological when an additional factor intrudes to inhibit the cognitive process of griefwork from running its course. This factor could be excessive drug use, alcohol use, or psychosis—but, most frequently, it is self-blame. This prevents the sadness produced by a loss from being resolved in its natural, timely way. And, when that inhibiting factor is self-reproach, it also adds feelings of worthlessness, self-hate, and a much more pronounced tendency to suicide to the list of the person's clinical symptoms—which thereby transforms his regular grief into a genuine, pathological depression. A complete anhedonia, in fact, need not be present for this kind of depression; although, if the thing that was lost was supremely important to the person, it certainly can be.

When it comes to therapy, there are three different paths to curing a first episode of major depression produced by a loss in the past. The patient can (1) reevaluate the loss itself, (2) reevaluate his self-reproach (when that's the inhibiting factor), or (3) regain or replace the thing that was lost. Using my own case as an example, let us examine these three possibilities.

We've already seen how, in the case of the fifteen-year-old me, my depression was dissolved instantly upon reevaluating the loss itself. I discovered that I truly had been to blame for the loss, but that it actually wasn't a loss at all. And what a profoundly amazing cure!

To have the tenacious, debilitating, and even life-threatening malady of depression cast off in a single mental event is, in a way, the holy grail of psychological cures. In most cases, however, we can't expect any new information to convince a depressed person that whatever he lost wasn't important, or that it wasn't a loss at all—since, most of the time, it objectively was of great value to him. If that's so, the person must travel a different path to the cure.

A second option is reevaluating his self-reproach over the actual fact of the loss. This won't instantly cure his depression, like the first path, but it will remove his impediment to consciously processing it—and allow him to actively reevaluate his loss in the organic, gradual way one adjusts to the death of a loved one. This path to recovery, clearly, takes much more time than the first option, and leaves the person to suffer more of the harmful effects of a prolonged, stressful period of sadness. For most cases of depression produced by a loss in the past, however, directly reevaluating the loss isn't possible, while reevaluating one's self-blame (in one way or another) can be achieved in practically all situations. The attainment of closure may be instrumental in either path to the cure.

A third path to the cure is a physical, instead of a psychological one. It requires the person to regain or replace the thing that was lost. This is, in fact, the instinctual cure to depression. If, for example, a person's depression is caused by an immature breakup, beginning a new relationship will dissolve his depression instantly. He will cease being tormented by what he let slip away, since he's now as well off as he was then, and quit brooding over the history of his former relationship, to become fully and eagerly absorbed with the details of the new one. That this type of replacement is, in such cases, the natural remedy for depression is indicated by the fact that it's precisely what the depressed person seeks and yearns for—often, it is the only thing he yearns for.

A Loss in the Future

A loss in the future, to produce a depression, must be the loss of a plan, expectation, or hope (whether conscious or unconscious) upon which one's ability to project a gratifying future for oneself depends. As John Stuart Mill said of his main goal in life, the (temporary) loss of which caused his depression: "All my happiness was to have been found in the continual pursuit of this end." The depressions produced by this type of loss typically, if not always, include anhedonia, but only rarely exhibit self-blame (except in people already predisposed to it, who consistently blame themselves for everything). That's because it's frequently difficult to determine what exactly the person lost, or how. There's also rarely an obvious, concrete event for which the person can blame himself, or which he can pinpoint as being the moment of his life-shattering loss.

The provoking event is, in most cases, an internal one—obtaining some new information, having a realization, or coming to a conclusion that throws one's whole view of the future into shambles. Or, if there is an external event, it's usually some trivial or ephemeral one that indirectly leads the person to this type of knowledge, conclusion, or realization. (The recurrent episodes of major depression resulting from rumination are always the product of this type of loss. They're always caused by a loss in the future, when—without anything happening—the chronic depressive manages to convince himself that his future is hopeless, his efforts are pointless, and all of his goals and ambitions are naïve illusions he'll never reach.)

In some cases, however, a loss in the future can be the result of a major, legitimate life-event. Examples include: Not getting into one's college of choice; being rejected by a potential lover; having a book, art project, or start-up one expectantly worked on meet with a disappointing reception; or even completing some central mission in life, only to find that one doesn't have anything left to strive for. In these cases, the resultant depression can clearly contain self-reproach, which then adds another complicating factor.

The cure for a first Major Depressive Episode caused by a loss in the future is also a reevaluation, but of a somewhat different nature. The first step is, of course, to identify what has been lost and how—which is already to travel half the path to the cure. Then, depending on what one discovers, the remedy can take multiple different forms.

Sometimes, a person will truly have lost his main goal, purpose, or aspiration in life, making his future appear like a barren wasteland. This may be caused by some new knowledge or understanding of the world, which makes him see that his goal's unattainable, that it won't bring him happiness even if he attained it, or that it is—fundamentally—immoral or evil. It can also be the result of a genuine life-event, like being rejected from one's college of choice, which makes the future one had envisioned physically impossible. Or it might be the consequence of, at long last, successfully completing one's previous mission in life, deriving whatever satisfaction one could from it, but then being left with no meaningful thing to pursue (losing one's purpose in life by means of completing it). In all of these cases, the cure lies in restructuring your idea of the future; finding a new goal, pursuit, or plan for your life that is both realistic and satisfying; and in this way projecting a new, positive future for yourself that you can look forward to. (This is, at the same time, a reevaluation and a replacement.)[79]

---

[79] This kind of depression is often a useful, important turning point in a person's life. Surprisingly often, I've heard people describe the main narrative of their life in this way: "I was on such and such path in life (usually set by their parents, or some misguided assumptions, or one they just fell into accidentally) and pursued it diligently, successfully, and without much questioning. Then, I realized that all that success wasn't making me happy, and getting more of it never would. At that point, I got extremely depressed, which I now see was a great blessing. It led me to find what I *really* wanted to do with my life, and now I am happily, passionately, and successfully doing *that*." In such instances, depression provides a much-needed pause, forcing the person to withdraw from a way of being that wasn't working, find his bearings, and change course for a new and superior direction.

Sometimes, however, the loss in the future is of a different kind. Rather than losing his main goal in life outright, some new information, realization, or disappointment may show the person that his projected timeline or magnitude for success at that goal—along with the whole view of the future he built around it—was overly optimistic, and (given what he's just learned) will not possibly occur as expected. This is a fairly common scenario. In that case, the cure lies in adjusting his expectations within this new context, accepting that his life won't be as great as imagined, and proceeding forward on the same path, but with a humbler, more tempered, more realistic view of the future.

And sometimes, it is the person's *conclusion* that the future he anticipated has been lost that's actually erroneous, shortsighted, or based on incomplete information. When that is the case, although the person might not realize this, recovery lies in obtaining some new information or understanding of the world that corrects his mistaken conclusion. Then, the person will see that his depression and hopelessness was based on a false premise, and can go back to living his life as before.

In cases where there's an inhibiting factor—whether it's drugs, alcohol, or self-blame—removing that factor, in whatever manner, will clearly facilitate the person's recovery.

(In John Stuart Mill's case, the loss in the future that caused his depression was really a mix of all three possibilities. His conclusion—that his mission in life would not bring him happiness—had been mistaken, but only partially. The *real* crisis in his projected future was, instead, of the second variety: that pursuing his primary "object in life" would *not* make him miserable, yet would not make him as happy as he expected. He also concluded "that the flaw in my life, [was also] a flaw in life itself," and if he did fully succeed in reforming society and government, so that "every person in the community were free and in a state of physical comfort, the pleasures of life," which could only be "kept up by struggle and privation, would cease to be pleasures." His main goal in life was, by that reasoning, a false goal: a dead end not worthy of pursuing. His cure came with the realization that "there was real, permanent happiness" to be gained in "poetry" and "in tranquil contemplation"—which would, in fact, "be made richer by every improvement in the physical or social condition of mankind." Seeing that, he was "never again subject" to his "habitual depression," and continued pursuing the same exact course for his life—perhaps slightly altered to incorporate reading some poetry—being now reassured of his goal's rectitude, but expecting less satisfaction from it than he did earlier.)

A Loss in the Present

A loss in the present is a lot like a loss in the past, but one with a highly pronounced, negative impact on one's current living conditions—making the actual circumstances one has to live under extremely unpleasant, stressful, or even unbearable. It also, in most cases, involves a loss in the future—making this type of loss the most difficult of all.[80]

My present-day girlfriend, for instance, ended up withdrawing from college in the first half of her senior year as a result of a Major Depressive Episode brought on by rumination, which precipitated a suicide attempt. She spent the next three weeks in a mental health clinic, during which time she didn't attend classes, lost both the jobs she was working at to earn money, and fell a month behind on paying her rent. After a conversation with her college advisor, she agreed to withdraw from the academic semester, and return home.

In a perfect example of the way that depression deepens and perpetuates depression, and how a Major Depressive Episode— even one brought on by rumination—can lead a person to make catastrophic decisions that have the potential to ruin his life, my girlfriend found herself back from her forty-thousand dollar a year

---

[80] Those whose depression was caused by this type of loss—or any loss involving a future dimension—commonly describe feeling "trapped" by their circumstances, having no way out of their current position into a future they can enjoy.

university in California, to her mother's apartment in the government projects where she had grown up. A major loss in the past,
present, and future: her depression now spanned all three dimensions.

Not only had she lost her previous, more-or-less happy life, with
best friends and intellectual challenges in an idyllic, luxurious campus
in California. Not only did she lose her whole bright, positive vision
of the future, including finishing college with a prestigious degree,
and receiving a well-paying job she enjoyed doing. But, perhaps
worst of all, she was now living again in the New York City ghetto,
with the narcissist mother who used to abuse her, having no money,
income, and a towering student loan debt, and seeing fresh bullet
holes in the door to the stairs in her hallway, just a few feet outside
her own door, where (as she told me) a young black man was shot
dead only a few days before her return.

The cure for this type of depression, therefore, has to span all
three fronts. My girlfriend, for example, not only needed to process
and come to peace with the event that caused the catastrophe. She
not only needed to modify her idea of the future, make a new plan
for herself, and set a humbler, more tempered, more realistic timeline
for her success. She also needed to physically fix the stressful, op-
pressive, nearly unbearable circumstances of her present life, making
them at least partially bearable and less stressful, as she worked to
accomplish the new future she laid out for herself, where she escaped
her current living conditions completely for a better, successful, and
enjoyable lifestyle. This final part is, in most cases, by far the most
difficult, since while the past and the future dimensions of this type
of loss have to be solved psychologically, at the speed of thought, its
present dimension has to be solved physically, at the speed of action,
which usually takes a lot longer. In my girlfriend's case, this last step
took almost ten years. (I'm happy to say, however, that she succeeded—with a little bit of my help—and is now a highly paid soft-
ware developer in California at a job that she loves.)

Hers wasn't, of course, a *first* Major Depressive Episode, but the
basic principles remain the same. A first Major Depressive Episode,

too, can be caused by a loss that affects all three dimensions, and has to be overcome by a remedy that addresses all three. To give a hypothetical example: A woman's first episode of major depression can be produced by the death of her husband, which leaves her to care for two school-aged children all on her own. To recover from her depression, then, she has to (1) successfully grieve and make peace with the death of her husband, (2) let go of her previous vision of the future, in which her husband played an integral role, and form a new, reassessed plan for her life that is both realistic and gratifying, and (3) adjust to the new, burdensome conditions of her present life; or drastically change those conditions by her own actions (essentially adjusting them to herself); or even flee from those grueling circumstances entirely, if that is at all possible.

To escape hopelessness, depression, and anhedonia, after all, a person needs to envision a future in which she'll be happy, and which she can actually achieve. Before she can go on to pursue that future, however, she must first overcome the current catastrophe that her loss in the present (by definition) has thrust upon her. Usually, this involves a straightforward process of adaptation, of gradually adjusting and learning to live, or even thrive, in the new situation life has imposed on you. The newly-made widow, to use our example, may see her future fulfillment and happiness in a certain career path. But to efficiently pursue that path, she must first figure out life as a single mother, find a way to feed, raise, and care for her two children without her dead husband's help, and to manage all this while still having time to pursue her own goals. In some cases, however, adjusting herself to the present conditions will simply be incompatible with achieving a future where she can be happy. Perhaps to support and take care of her kids, the widow must pause her career plans for over a decade, working some menial job close to home that she greatly dislikes, and which she can tell is too stressful and burdensome for her to sustain without being overcome by depression. (And high levels of stress are, as we know, a depressed person's natural enemy.) She must then drastically change her physical situation, perhaps sending her kids off to boarding school, or having them live half the time with a relative, or rapidly finding a new man to marry who will help her take care of them. If even that is impossible, however, the only way to escape her depression might be to escape her present conditions entirely—perhaps giving her kids up to foster care, or to a friend, relative, or whoever will take them—and going off to continue her life independently, pursuing a future she can actually bear. (Although such a choice may appear heartless, it is certainly better—for both her and her kids—than the alternative of being consumed by depression, which would make her unable to take care of her kids anyway, or even induce her to commit suicide, which would clearly be worse still.)

Aleksandr Solzhenitsyn escaped his depression in precisely this way: by physically fleeing his home in Soviet Russia—where he feared being arrested at any moment—to a secret hiding place in Estonia, where the KGB wasn't aware of his presence, and where he continued his work on his primary mission in life (which was writing the *Gulag Archipelago*).

Chapter 13

Sadness in Animals

It is adapting to the real-life consequences of a loss in the present that seems to be the main evolutionary function of the emotion of sadness. Most higher animals (including dogs, wolves, apes, geese, dolphins, magpies, and elephants) exhibit a grief response at the death of a close individual, and most likely for that exact reason.

Animals don't have explicit memories of the past, and they don't have any plans for the future. What they do have are behaviors, reactions, and learned expectations adjusted to a certain environment. When that environment changes, like when a close individual that was a large part of that environment—be it a mate, friend, parent, or offspring—dies, the animal will feel sad, apparently as a way to untie its learned expectations of pleasure and reward from certain behaviors centered on that individual, and replace them with new behaviors and expectations better suited to its altered environment.

C.S. Lewis wrote of his grief after the death of his wife, that it involved "the frustration of so many impulses that had become habitual. Thought after thought, feeling after feeling, action after action, had [his wife] for their object. Now their target is gone. I keep on through habit fitting an arrow to the string, then I remember and have to lay the bow down." This is, indeed, the way sadness helps us (and animals) adapt to the practical consequences of a loss in the present.

For humans, just as in animals, our actions are orchestrated almost entirely by the pleasure principle (an instinctual compulsion to increase pleasure and reduce displeasure). Before engaging in any activity, we first anticipate that activity in our minds, creating a mental representation of it, which carries associations of pleasure and displeasure—associations unconsciously (and inextricably) based on our actual experience of it in reality. If we anticipate a net gain in pleasure (or decrease in displeasure) from a certain activity, we are motivated to engage in it, and are willing to expend effort in order to do so. If we anticipate a net loss of pleasure (or increase in displeasure) from that activity, we are motivated in the opposite way, and are willing to expend effort in order to avoid it.

Normally, our day-to-day adaptation to our current environment consists of having a range of available activities we've learned to obtain pleasure and relieve displeasure through. Often, many of these activities involve a person (and sometimes an object, and sometimes a job) that has been extensively integrated into our lives. These may include hugging, kissing, confiding in, complaining at, watching a movie with, buying small presents for, or talking on the phone to one's husband or wife. The pangs of sadness evoked by the memory of this recently lost person add a weight of displeasure to thoughts of all such potential activities, making our associations to them net pleasure-negative, and demotivating us from pursuing them.

This works on a purely neurological, associative level, tacking on painful displeasure to automatic associations of pleasure, and thereby extinguishing our learned expectations of a reward in a changed environment that can no longer provide it. This holds equally true for the child whose mother died, the husband whose wife divorced him, and the dog whose owner abandoned it. In both humans and animals, grief prunes our associative network of pleasurable expectations, by pairing our previous anticipations of pleasure with the painful emotion of sadness. (The fact that sadness also motivates humans to consciously process a loss in the past, and find some meaning in it, or analyze a loss in the future, and discover the cause of it, is only a later evolutionary development—a highly common occurrence in evolution, in which a previously evolved mechanism is adapted to serve a new function.)

Chapter 14

Depression in Animals

But animals also experience depression—both of the chronic and single episode varieties. And just like in humans, these are set off by intense stressors. Animals, of course, don't have explicit memories, or ruminate, or construct plans for the future. Their primary source of acute stress, then, is their physical environment, some real-life calamity that they have to live through, and which places them under significant stress. This is, at minimum, analogous to a loss in the present—but usually, and possibly always, it literally *is* a loss in the present that produces animal depression.

Psychologists have identified at least two types of losses that reliably cause depression in animals. One is the loss of status, the other's the loss of a mother (or a temporary loss in the form of a separation) early in life.

Rhesus monkeys briefly separated from their mothers in childhood exhibit a pattern of depression very similar to that of humans. Experiments demonstrate that, upon separation, the young monkeys become passive, cry, and show a huge increase in self-grooming, self-rocking, and other self-soothing behaviors. After a limited time, the monkeys are reunited with their mothers, and grow up to become more or less like the other, never-separated monkeys. But when exposed to a major stressor in adulthood, specifically a brief social isolation, they react very differently from the normal monkeys:

exhibiting the same depressive behaviors of inactivity, crying, and different types of self-soothing. The more times they were separated from their mothers in childhood, the more intense their depressive reactions were in adulthood; and the more times they were subjected to social isolation during adulthood, the more intense their depressive reactions were on the next isolation. These early-life separations seem analogous to the ACEs (adverse childhood experiences) of humans, while their adult reactions to isolation seem analogous to Major Depressive Episodes.

Status, and one's rank in the dominance hierarchy of the individuals one competes with, plays a crucial (if often overlooked) role in the lives of animals from every end of the evolutionary spectrum—including most primates, wolves, birds, and even (as Jordan Peterson points out) lobsters. An animal, to survive and reproduce, has to compete with other animals for limited resources—for food, water, shelter, and (very importantly) members of the opposite sex. In species that form dominance hierarchies, this competition takes place by means of literal, physical fighting—at least in the last resort. Male baboons, for example, will physically take food, shelter, and females from smaller, weaker baboons, and attack them violently if they protest. In the animal kingdom, force rules, and might most emphatically equals right. But actual battle is dangerous and costly, even for the stronger opponent, who despite gaining victory, can himself sustain serious injuries. To avoid violent combat, therefore, these animals evolved ways to assess their own fighting ability, and that of others, and to predict the outcome of a battle without actually battling.

They do this by forming dominance hierarchies, by ranking themselves and those who they live and compete with by order of physical strength. Such rank is established and maintained by various "dominance interactions," such as aggressive vocalizing, bearing one's teeth, non-violent or ritualized combat (like rough play or wrestling, in which the animals test one another's strength), and—only as a very last resort—actual fighting. The brain of these animals (in one way or another) registers and stores the outcome of these interactions, by which they implicitly understand their position in the hierarchy, and which they acknowledge to one another through gestures of dominance and submission. (In baboons, for example, the weaker monkey, whether male or female, will turn around and "present" its backside—placing itself in a helpless, vulnerable position—in front of a stronger monkey, acknowledging its dominance; while the stronger monkey, whether male or female, will briefly climb on its back and "mount" it, or brush its genitals with the back of its hand—all in a purely nonsexual way—thus acknowledging the other's submission.)

At the top of the hierarchy, the strongest, most dominant, alpha baboon, wolf, or lobster (who can defeat all the others in battle) has access to all the best food, shelter, and females. Next up, the second-rank, beta animal (who can defeat all but the first rank in battle) has access to all the best resources not claimed by the alpha. The third-ranker, who can defeat all but the alpha and beta, has access to all the best resources not claimed by them—and so on and so forth, all down the line. An animal's place in the dominance hierarchy, therefore, dictates nearly every detail of its day-to-day life, making a drop in its ranking a major, disastrous upheaval, which often produces an episode of depression across a variety of different species.

An alpha's position is so valuable that he will rarely relinquish it without fighting. The alpha baboon, for instance, defends his rank violently from all challengers. He's usually successful in fending them off, leaves them with gashes and injuries, and continues his reign as the top monkey. Eventually, however, the alpha grows older and weaker, while some upstart baboon grows bigger and stronger, violently battles him for the top rank, and overthrows him to become the new alpha. Toppled, the old alpha—frequently, but not always—falls into an overt depression. He becomes passive, hangs his head, and sits far away from the other monkeys. But not only that.

There is, to use Jordan Peterson's words, an ancient *dominance calculator* in the animal's brain: what other authors consider a primitive "self-concept" of its fighting capacity, and which they think "may be the evolutionary primordium of human self-esteem" (something I tend to agree with). This ancient dominance calculator regulates a wide range of the animal's behavior, internal biology, and even its external morphology. The overthrown alpha baboons, their dominance counter recording their loss of status, not only acted depressed: within weeks they lost body mass, the reddish sexual skin of their face had turned grey, and the dense hair of their majestic mantels (another sexual feature) had fallen out. A dominant lobster defeated in battle not only appears sullen, and refrains—for a time— from fighting even those weaker than him: the neurological circuitry of its brain physically restructures itself, transforming into the brain of a subordinate lobster, one better suited to fleeing from conflict than engaging in battle. All of these are, of course, understandable and adaptive changes: The former alpha baboons, who in losing their status also lost all of their females, ceased spending resources to maintain their secondary sexual characteristics, which became useless to them in their new environment; and the defeated lobsters, no longer the strongest ones in their territory, had to become better at fleeing to avoid damage.

The monkeys' reactions to social defeat, complete with reduced self-esteem, significant weight loss, and diminished sexual interest (all characteristic of human depression), are clearly analogous to single episodes of major depression—and oftentimes first episodes, in monkeys that never exhibited this type of reaction before. Lose enough dominance battles, however, and your rank will continue to drop, and so will your dominance counter, until the monkey, or wolf, or whatever creature you are, falls to the very-most bottom of the dominance hierarchy. And that is where chronic depression resides. The lowest ranking baboon, for example, closely resembles a chronically depressed human: The creature is constantly anxious and jittery, downcast and withdrawn, sleeps intermittently, eats very little, has practically no sex drive, is extremely reactive to tiny quantities of stress, and its hormone levels, impaired immune functioning, and the "constellation of changes" in its brain biochemistry are the same as those found in chronically depressed humans.

Jordan Peterson makes a highly compelling case for this being, in fact, an evolved adaptation to life at the bottom of the dominance hierarchy—using "those who exist on the lower rungs of [human] society" as an example. These people are broke, they "have nowhere to live (or nowhere good)," their "food is terrible, when they're not going hungry," they're in poor physical shape, they have no reliable friends, and they're "of minimal romantic interest" to anybody. Possessing no store of resources to fall back on—neither physical, like money or health insurance; nor personal, like marketable skills or even good social skills; nor interpersonal, like a supportive family, or friends, or even a religious community—what might be a small inconvenience for most other people, can be an unmitigated disaster to those on the fringes of human society. In this context, extreme stress reactivity is a useful trait: "You need that reactivity," writes Jordan Peterson, because "emergencies are common at the bottom." Even in the face of a minor stressor, this person "must be prepared to do anything and everything, in case it becomes necessary," since the smallest of hazards might set off "an uncontrollable chain of negative events, which will have to be handled alone."[81]

---

[81] This is why, in the landmark study of depression in women living in a working-class London suburb, a supportive husband reduced the chance of contracting depression in the wake of a major stressor by 75 percent (from four-in-ten to one-out-of-ten), compared to the women who had no social support. A safety net of this sort makes major life stressors, well, a whole lot less stressful. It not only mitigates crises when they occur, preventing depression caused by a loss in the present; it's also especially helpful for chronic depressives, preventing depression resulting from rumination.

With the ability to anticipate the future, a human is able to brood upon, worry about, and stress out over potential disasters that only *might* happen to him. And as a rule, the stress he feels from imagining a future disaster will be proportional—perhaps exaggerated, perhaps underestimated, but *proportional*—to the magnitude of the potential disaster. In chronic depressives, of course, merely anticipating a crisis can spiral down (by way of rumination) into a full-blown major depression, without the crisis itself actually happening, since the person convinces himself it's inevitable. A safety net in the form of a supportive husband (or

This would explain why a couple episodes of major depression can produce such profound changes in the human brain: Because there's already an ancient, depressive mode our brain can go into, the potential for which has evolved over millions of years—a state of extreme stress reactivity, depressed mood, and zero self-esteem—expressly adapted (at least in our primate ancestors) for life at the bottom of the dominance hierarchy. It's tempting to think that, in the monkeys with chronic depression produced by an early-life separation from their mothers, their brains also enter this mode because they are the monkeys most likely—due to the large impact good mothering has on later-life thriving—to wind up being the bottom rankers.

Very interestingly, points out Jordan Peterson, the dominance calculator in lobsters is regulated by serotonin: the neurotransmitter also deeply involved, but in a much more complex way, in the dominance (or self-esteem) feelings of mice, monkeys, humans, and—in all likelihood—every creature in between. In lobsters, the mechanism is highly rudimentary. Winning a dominance battle increases the serotonin in its bloodstream. Losing a dominance battle decreases the serotonin in its blood stream. Giving a lobster Prozac after it loses a dominance battle (a human antidepressant that acts to increase serotonin levels), will erase the effects of that loss, and make the crustacean ready to hop into battle again, as if nothing happened.

---

friends, or family, or a religious community), who the depressive knows she can count on if things go wrong, also reduces the magnitude of *possible* crises, and thereby effectively prevents even depressions resulting from rumination.

When I saw these statistics and apprehended this point, I knew I had to follow the data. The best thing I could do for my depressive girlfriend, I realized, was to *be* this kind of safety net for her (if only temporarily). That is what I did, and it likely contributed to her present success.

Chapter 15

Drugs

Having dissected the causes and cures of various types of depression, it's time we revisited the topic of medication, and discussed the role it can play in treating this malady.

Antidepressants

Richard O'Connor draws an important distinction: Depressed people, he says, have "symptoms," and then they have "problems." Antidepressants can alleviate the symptoms, and make the patient more able to tackle his problems. First, let's take a look at the way medication can reduce symptoms.

There are, as we know, dozens of different antidepressants, all of them with more-or-less different effects, and which are furthermore different for each person. When they work, however, they seem to produce their beneficial effects by modulating the intensity of certain affects. By simply making the same stimulus produce a different intensity of emotional response, these drugs can profoundly alter a person's behavior and personality.

Prozac, and the other antidepressant drugs of its class (the Selective Serotonin Reuptake Inhibitors), are known to reduce "rejection sensitivity"—the painful emotions a person feels in response to a loss, rejection, or disappointment (whether real or anticipated).

This makes them remarkably resilient in the face of real setbacks, and lets them take risks that they otherwise wouldn't dare to. It also appears to take much of the sting out of the numerous, tiny difficulties of social interaction—and often transforms insecure, socially inhibited people into outgoing, gregarious individuals. Other varieties of antidepressants can enhance the happiness or excitement a person feels in response to positive events; others can make him feel less agitated and anxious; while others may diminish his baseline sadness. By simply tweaking a few dials on the intensity of his emotional responses (even if completely at random), these drugs can genuinely alter a person's experience of living. They may, of course, have terrible side effects, and change that experience for the worse. Sometimes, however, they will change the patient's experience for the better, and if not turn him into a more-or-less functional and content person, at least get him out of his current mental and behavioral rut, so he can go about solving the problems that underlie his depression.

Antidepressants are chronic, long-term, personality-altering drugs. They take four to eight weeks to kick in, and are meant to be taken indefinitely. They're clearly a long-term solution to a long-term problem. The distinction between chronic depression, and the three types of first Major Depressive Episode set off by a loss in the past, present, or future, is highly significant here. A first episode caused by a loss in the past or the future is obviously a poor candidate for antidepressant treatment. These types, as we saw, call for a psychological cure, which can be achieved rather rapidly through conscious analysis. Chronic depression, on the other hand, is the best candidate for antidepressants—a persistent, potentially lifelong condition, which the person must struggle with and resist while resolving his many practical and psychological problems. Antidepressants can lighten his burden, diminish his symptoms, and make his lengthy ordeal—of obtaining the necessities for psychological health—a lot easier. A first episode caused by a loss in the present inhabits a middle ground. It also requires solving a long-term practical problem—though typically only a single, central one like finishing college, obtaining employment, or earning enough money to fund an important goal—which can take many months or years. But in such cases, where the central problem is primarily work-related, a stimulant such as Adderall (a drug that improves focus and allows people to work doggedly at difficult and largely unpleasant tasks) can be a much better alternative—given its immediate action, predictability, and specificity of effect. (And I've known several people for whom this was the case.) Still, when the central problem is mainly social, like gaining new friends, finding a romantic partner, or mending one's existing relationships, antidepressants may indeed be the best option.

Psychedelics

There is, however, a different class of drugs that are highly effective where antidepressants aren't. These are the so-called psychedelic drugs. Psychedelic means "mind revealing," which refers to these drugs' potential to show a person parts of his mind he normally couldn't (or didn't want to) examine. Unlike antidepressants, these are short-term, fast-acting, consciousness-altering drugs. They last from four to twelve hours, depending on the drug, and have their beneficial effects not by regulating people's brain chemistry, but through the new, powerful experiences people frequently have while taking them.

The classic psychedelic drugs include mescaline (the active ingredient in peyote cactus), psilocybin (the active ingredient in magic mushrooms), LSD, DMT, and MDMA. Although, as of 2019, these drugs are illegal almost everywhere in the world, they are rapidly gaining both popular and official recognition as powerful tools for therapy and psychological growth. Psilocybin (the active ingredient in magic mushrooms) has just received "breakthrough therapy status" in the United States for treating treatment-resistant depression. MDMA received the same "breakthrough therapy status" for treating Post-Traumatic Stress Disorder. And ketamine (a different psychedelic that can be legally administered in a medical setting) has for several years now been used for treating depression, and with success rates that blow antidepressants out of the water.

While working on this book, I had the chance to try psychedelics, and I can attest: they are extremely powerful drugs, with enormous potential as agents for therapeutic change. Almost every hour in psychotherapy is spent on trying to get around the patient's defenses: his defenses against change, against understanding, against honestly admitting his problems. And all psychedelics have this one thing in common: they chemically inactivate the regions of the brain responsible for a person's defenses. As consciousness-altering drugs, they alter the functionality of a person's mental apparatus, amplifying some parts of it, while shutting down others, but leaving him highly lucid, rational, and clearheaded throughout. This allows him to observe certain parts of his psyche in isolation from the rest, which can let him directly access and identify the exact causes of his psychological troubles. The experiences people have on these drugs include grand realizations; confrontations with past trauma; reassessments of old beliefs; new gains in self-knowledge; intimate connections with nature, or one's own being, or other people; and extremely acute, even transcendent, periods of pleasure, ecstasy, bliss (what Abraham Maslow called peak-experiences). At the very least, they can grant the user an on-demand moment of lucidity (at some point during, or possibly after, the experience), in which he can coldly, dispassionately examine his problems, and obtain a wider, unemotional, bird's-eye-view perspective on them—something most depressed people vitally need.

Exactly the opposite of antidepressants, psychedelics are most fit for treating a first Major Depressive Episode produced by a loss in the past or the future, which can often be cured by a single realization, and which is precisely what these drugs provide best. They can likewise resolve the past and the future dimensions of a first episode caused by a loss in the present, and even greatly speed up the process of readjustment to the practical consequences of that loss. Chronic depression is the worst match for psychedelic drugs, but then again, it's not a good match for any available treatment. An interwoven tangle of practical, psychological, and neurochemical problems, it can't be cured by a one-shot psychological event (like first episodes that only have future or past dimensions), nor by the skyhook of some fortunate real-world event, like suddenly finding a new job or relationship (which might instantly cure a first episode cause by a loss in the present).

Rather than any single event, the cure for chronic depression must be an upward spiral: a lengthy process of growth taking multiple months or years, in which the person resolves his practical and psychological problems faster than they pull him down into depression. Psychedelics, which only last half a day and shouldn't be taken more than once every few weeks, clearly can't ease this process like antidepressants can. What they can do, however, is *initiate* the upward spiral, and which by all indications is the way psilocybin—the active ingredient in magic mushrooms that just received breakthrough therapy status in the US for treating treatment-resistant depression—sometimes cures chronic depressions too.

At the higher doses at which it is most effective, psilocybin can generate ecstatic, acutely pleasurable peak-experiences, one taste of which can prevent suicide for a lifetime. The mere knowledge that something so positive is possible (and rather easily attainable) is sufficient to give someone, especially the depressed person who thinks he'll never experience pleasure again, a real reason to continue living and bettering himself—which can certainly jumpstart an upward spiral. And although psilocybin's period of action (a few hours every several weeks or months) doesn't nearly cover the time a person must struggle with chronic depression, its efficacy as a treatment—at least according to the preliminary data—is much higher than antidepressants, and it often succeeds in the cases where antidepressants fail.

Psychedelics, however, have their own dangers as well. Although most of them are non-addictive, and do not produce physical dependency, some of them—especially ketamine, and to a lesser extent MDMA—do carry that risk. They can also notoriously lead to what have been called "bad trips:" prolonged periods not of acute pleasure and ecstasy, but horror and despair, a taste not of heaven, but of hell, which may sometimes prove highly valuable, but more often result in real psychological trauma. When taken with professional supervision and in a therapeutic setting, however, bad trips can be easily avoided and their risk reduced nearly to zero. Perhaps most importantly, psychedelics shouldn't be mixed with antidepressants, since the chemical interaction between some psychedelics and some antidepressants can actually prove fatal. In other cases, one psychedelic session can sabotage the already established positive influence of an antidepressant, which rests on maintaining a precarious chemical balance in the person's brain, and might render him no longer responsive to that particular medication.

That last point, however, is more an indictment of antidepressants than psychedelics, since being dependent on them disqualifies the psychedelic option, which often can be a much better choice. This will, I think, become a serious issue for antidepressant use in the next decades, as psychedelic-assisted therapy becomes a widespread and legalized treatment for mental illness.

Chapter 16

The Introspective Microscope

I have frequently said that diagnosis of mental illness today is much like the diagnosis of physical illness was in medieval times, before the microscope had been invented. Doctors still could identify diseases: collections of symptoms that typically occurred together, which appeared to be caused by exposure to certain conditions, and which ran a fairly predictable course from contraction to recovery. The only problem was, nobody knew why, or how, these diseases occurred. Only with the invention of the microscope, could people finally observe the microbes responsible for their illnesses, along with their method of action in the human body.

Psychologists who examine the behavior, symptoms, and self-reports of others, but ignore their own mental processes as scientifically valid data, are like medieval physicians who had microscopes, but threw them away. Introspection is the microscope of psychology: the power to directly observe in yourself the psychological processes you can only infer in others. And much like a physical microscope, it grants you invaluable access to a different, deeper level of knowledge about the nature of reality, a human's internal reality, that can't be acquired in any other way.

It's certainly true that the one mind you can introspectively observe is your own, and you are the only person who can observe that mind, which presents a real obstacle for observers in pursuit of agreement about some aspect of human psychology. But this isn't an insurmountable obstacle, not by a long shot.

In this book, I applied my introspective microscope to the problem of depression. And I hope I have shown how knowledge attained in this way can be enormously useful for understanding, and ultimately freeing ourselves, from the psychological troubles that burden our lives.

Your Free Bonus Essay!

Congratulations, you've made it to the end of this book!

As a token of thanks, I'd like to give you access to Sigmund Freud's foundational essay on *Mourning and Melancholia*, free of charge.

Freud's essay provides some strikingly brilliant insights into the psychology of depression. It had essentially launched the psychological study of depression early in the twentieth century, and is a highly recommended complement to this book.

To download the essay, just visit:

www.romangelperin.com/freudpdf

You'll also have an opportunity to receive exclusive access to my newest books, free books, and other valuable messages from me.

———

To Learn More about the Author, please visit:

www.RomanGelperin.com

or send him an
email at

romangelperin@gmail.com

———

Thank you for Reading

Works Cited

American Psychiatric Association. *Diagnostic and Statistical Manual of Mental Disorders: DSM-5.* Arlington, Va., American Psychiatric Association, 2013.

---. *Diagnostic and Statistical Manual of Mental Disorders: DSM-IV-TM.* Washington, American Psychiatric Association, 2005.

---. "Highlights of Changes from DSM-IV-TR to DSM-5." 2013. https://www.mirecc.va.gov/VISN16/docs/APA_DSM_4_to_5_Changes.pdf. Accessed May 2019.

Arieti, Silvano, and Jules Bemporad. *Severe and Mild Depression: The Psychotherapeutic Approach.* Digital Edition. International Psychotherapy Institute eBooks, 2014, www.freepsychotherapybooks.org/ebook/severe-and-mild-depression. Accessed 4 May 2019.

Beck, Aaron, and Brad Alford. *Depression: Causes and Treatment.* Philadelphia, University of Pennsylvania Press, 2009.

Beck, Aaron, and Sigmund Valin. "Psychotic Depressive Reactions in Soldiers Who Accidentally Killed Their Buddies." *American Journal of Psychiatry*, vol. 110, no. 5, Nov. 1953, pp. 347–353, 10.1176/ajp.110.5.347.

Berg, Lisa, et al. "Parental Death during Childhood and Depression in Young Adults - a National Cohort Study." *Journal of Child Psychology and Psychiatry*, vol. 57, no. 9, 5 Apr. 2016, pp. 1092–1098, 10.1111/jcpp.12560.

Black, Donald W, et al. *DSM-5 Guidebook: The Essential Companion to the Diagnostic and Statistical Manual of Mental Disorders, Fifth Edition.* Washington, DC American Psychiatric Publishing, 2014.

Bowlby, John. *Attachment and Loss. Vol. 3 Loss, Sadness and Depression.* New York Basic Books, 1980.

Branden, Nathaniel. *Judgment Day : My Years with Ayn Rand.* Boston, Houghton Mifflin, 1989.

Brown, George W, et al. "Self-Esteem and Depression. 1. Measurement Issues and Prediction of Onset." *Social Psychiatry and Psychiatric Epidemiology*, vol. 25, no. 4, Jul. 1990, pp. 200–9, www.ncbi.nlm.nih.gov/pubmed/2399477.

Brown, George W. "Self-Esteem and Depression. III. Aetiological Issues." *Social Psychiatry and Psychiatric Epidemiology*, vol. 25, no. 5, Oct. 1990, pp. 235–43, www.ncbi.nlm.nih.gov/pubmed/2237604

Brown, George W, et al. "Social Support, Self-Esteem and Depression." *Psychological Medicine*, vol. 16, no. 04, Nov. 1986, p 813, journals.cambridge.org/abstract_S0033291700011831, 10.1017/s0033291700011831.

Brown, George W. "Psychosocial Factors and Depression and Anxiety Disorders- Some Possible Implications for Biological Research." *Journal of Psychopharmacology*, vol. 10, no. 1, Jan. 1996, pp. 23–30, 10.1177/026988119601000105.

Brown, George W, and Tirril O Harris. *Social Origins of Depression: A Study of Psychiatric Disorder in Women*. Abingdon, Oxfordshire; New York, Ny, Routledge, 2011.

Butler, Judith. *The Psychic Life of Power Theories in Subjection*. Stanford, Calif. Stanford Univ. Press, 1997.

Carhart-Harris, Robin L, et al. "Psilocybin with Psychological Support for Treatment-Resistant Depression: An Open-Label Feasibility Study." *The Lancet Psychiatry*, vol. 3, no. 7, Jul. 2016, pp. 619–627, 10.1016/s2215-0366(16)30065-7.

Casey, Nell. *Unholy Ghost: Writers on Depression*. New York, Harper Perennial, 2002.

Caspi, A. "Influence of Life Stress on Depression: Moderation by a Polymorphism in the 5-HTT Gene." *Science*, vol. 301, no. 5631, 18 July 2003, pp. 386–389, 10.1126/science.1083968.

Chapman, Daniel P., et al. "Adverse Childhood Experiences and the Risk of Depressive Disorders in Adulthood." *Journal of Affective Disorders*, vol. 82, no. 2, Oct. 2004, pp. 217–225, 10.1016/j.jad.2003.12.013.

Cheong, E Von, et al. "Adverse Childhood Experiences (ACEs) and Later-Life Depression: Perceived Social Support as a Potential Protective Factor." *BMJ Open*, vol. 7, no. 9, Sept. 2017, p. e013228, bmjopen.bmj.com/content/7/9/e013228, 10.1136/bmjopen-2016-013228.

Cochran, Susan D, et al. "Prevalence of Mental Disorders, Psychological Distress, and Mental Health Services Use among Lesbian, Gay, and Bisexual Adults in the United States." *Journal of Consulting and Clinical Psychology*, vol. 71, no. 1, Feb. 2003, pp. 53–61,
www.ncbi.nlm.nih.gov/pmc/articles/PMC4197971/.

DePaulo, Raymond, and Leslie Alan Horvitz. *Understanding Depression: What We Know and What You Can Do about It*. New York, Wiley, 2002.

Epstein, Seymour. *Constructive Thinking: The Key to Emotional Intelligence.* Westport, Conn., Praeger, 1998.

---. *Cognitive Experiental Theory : An Integrative Theory of Personality.* Oxford, Oxford University Press, 2014.

Freud, Sigmund. *Freud Complete Works.* Ivan Smith, 2000.

Freud, Sigmund, and Josef Breuer. *Studies on Hysteria.* New York, Basic Books, 2000.

Greenberg, Gary. *Manufacturing Depression: The Secret History of a Modern Disease.* Simon & Schuster, 2011.

Griffiths, R. R., et al. "Psilocybin Can Occasion Mystical-Type Experiences Having Substantial and Sustained Personal Meaning and Spiritual Significance." *Psychopharmacology*, vol. 187, no. 3, 7 July 2006, pp. 268–283, 10.1007/s00213-006-0457-5.

Hammen, Constance. *Depression.* Hove, Lawrence Erlbaum, 1997. books.google.com/books?id=9tY3gW3TAZkC

Hari, Johann. *Lost Connections: Uncovering the Real Causes of Depression.* New York, Bloomsbury, 2018.

Harlow, Harry F., and Stephen J. Suomi. "Induced Depression in Monkeys." *Behavioral Biology*, vol. 12, no. 3, Nov. 1974, pp. 273–296, 10.1016/s0091-6773(74)91475-8. Accessed 4 May 2019.

Harris, Sam. *Waking Up: A Guide to Spirituality without Religion.* New York, Simon & Schuster, 2014.

Heller, Anne C. *Ayn Rand and the World She Made.* New York, Anchor, 2010.

Jamison, Kay R. *Exuberance: The Passion for Life.* New York, Vintage Books, 2005.

Johnson, J, et al. "The Validity of Major Depression with Psychotic Features Based on a Community Study." *Archives of General Psychiatry*, vol. 48, no. 12, Dec. 1991, pp. 1075–81, www.ncbi.nlm.nih.gov/pubmed/1845225.

Karraa, Walker. *Transformed by Postpartum Depression: Women's Stories of Trauma and Growth.* Praeclarus Press, 2015.

Kendler, Kenneth S, et al. "A Swedish National Twin Study of Lifetime Major Depression." *The American Journal of Psychiatry*, vol. 163, no. 1, Jan. 2006, pp. 109–14, www.ncbi.nlm.nih.gov/pubmed/16390897, 10.1176/appi.ajp.163.1.109.

Kessler, R C, et al. "Comorbidity of DSM-III-R Major Depressive Disorder in the General Population: Results from the US

National Comorbidity Survey." *The British Journal of Psychiatry. Supplement*, no. 30, Jun. 1996, pp. 17–30, www.ncbi.nlm.nih.gov/pubmed/8864145.

Kessler, Ronald C. "Lifetime and 12-Month Prevalence of DSM-III-R Psychiatric Disorders in the United States." *Archives of General Psychiatry*, vol. 51, no. 1, 1 Jan. 1994, p. 8-19, jamanetwork.com/journals/jamapsychiatry/article-abstract/496456?redirect=true, 10.1001/archpsyc.1994.03950010008002.

---. "Lifetime Prevalence and Age-of-Onset Distributions of DSM-IV Disorders in the National Comorbidity Survey Replication." *Archives of General Psychiatry*, vol. 62, no. 6, 1 June 2005, p. 593, 10.1001/archpsyc.62.6.593.

Kummer, Hans. *In Quest of The Sacred Baboon: A Scientist's Journey.* Princeton University Press, 1995.

Lewis, C S. *A Grief Observed.* New York; Bantam, 1976.

Ma, S Helen, and John D Teasdale. "Mindfulness-Based Cognitive Therapy for Depression: Replication and Exploration of Differential Relapse Prevention Effects." *Journal of Consulting and Clinical Psychology*, vol. 72, no. 1, Feb. 2004, pp. 31–40, www.ncbi.nlm.nih.gov/pubmed/14756612, 10.1037/0022-006X.72.1.31.

Maj, M, et al. "Pattern of Recurrence of Illness after Recovery from an Episode of Major Depression: A Prospective Study." *The American Journal of Psychiatry*, vol. 149, no. 6, Jun. 1992, pp. 795–800, www.ncbi.nlm.nih.gov/pubmed/1590496, 10.1176/ajp.149.6.795.

Maslow, Abraham. *Motivation and Personality.* 3rd ed., Harper Collins Publishers, 1970.

---. *Religions, Values, and Peak-Experiences.* Penguin, 1970.

---. *Toward a Psychology of Being.* 2nd ed., New York, Van Nostrand, 1968.

Mill, John Stuart. "Autobiography of John Stuart Mill." *Project Gutenberg*, 2019, www.gutenberg.org/ebooks/10378.

Monroe, Scott M., et al. "Major Life Events and Major Chronic Difficulties Are Differentially Associated with History of Major Depressive Episodes." *Journal of Abnormal Psychology*, vol. 116, no. 1, 2007, pp. 116–124, www.ncbi.nlm.nih.gov/pmc/articles/PMC3631311/, 10.1037/0021-843x.116.1.116.

National Institute of Mental Health. "NIMH » Questions and Answers about the NIMH Sequenced Treatment Alternatives to Relieve Depression (STAR*D) Study — All Medication Levels." Nov. 2006. *Nih.Gov*, Accessed on 4 May, 2019, www.nimh.nih.gov/funding/clinical-research/practical/stard/allmedicationlevels.shtml.

O'Connor, Richard. *Undoing Depression: What Therapy Doesn't Teach You and Medication Can't Give You.* 2nd ed., New York, Ny, Little, Brown and Co, 2010.

---. *Undoing Perpetual Stress : The Missing Connection between Depression, Anxiety, and 21st Century Illness.* New York, Berkley Books, 2006.

Peterson, Jordan B. *12 Rules for Life: An Antidote to Chaos.* Penguin Books, 2019.

Pollan, Michael. *How to Change Your Mind: The New Science of Psychedelics.* Penguin Press, 2018.

Price, John, et al. "The Social Competition Hypothesis of Depression." *British Journal of Psychiatry*, vol. 164, no. 03, Mar. 1994, pp. 309–315, 10.1192/bjp.164.3.309.

Rand, Ayn. *Atlas Shrugged.* New York, Ny, Penguin Publishing Group, 1997.

Rei, Herbert E. *Depression in Childhood: A Survey of Some Pertinent Contributions.* 1996. www.jaacap.org/article/S0002-7138(09)61960-9/pdf

Samman, Josh. *The Housekeeper: Love, Death, and Prizefighting.* United States, Josh Samman, 2016.

Sapolsky, Robert M. *A Primate's Memoir: A Neuroscientist's Unconventional Life among the Baboons.* New York, Simon & Schuster, 2001.

---. *Why Zebras Don't Get Ulcers: The Acclaimed Guide to Stress, Stress-Related Diseases, and Coping.* New York, Henry Holt and Co, 2004.

Schalinski, Inga, et al. "Type and Timing of Adverse Childhood Experiences Differentially Affect Severity of PTSD, Dissociative and Depressive Symptoms in Adult Inpatients." *BMC Psychiatry*, vol. 16, no. 1, 19 Aug. 2016, 10.1186/s12888-016-1004-5.

Segal, Zindel V, et al. *Mindfulness-Based Cognitive Therapy for Depression.* Second Edition. New York; London, Guilford Press, 2013.

Solomon, Andrew. *The Noonday Demon: An Atlas of Depression.* New York, Scribner Classics, 2015.

Solomon, David A., et al. "Predicting Recovery from Episodes of Major Depression." *Journal of Affective Disorders*, vol. 107, no. 1–3, Apr. 2008, pp. 285–291, www.ncbi.nlm.nih.gov/pmc/articles/PMC2405955/, 10.1016/j.jad.2007.09.001.

---. "Recovery From Major Depression." *Archives of General Psychiatry*, vol. 54, no. 11, 1 Nov. 1997, p. 1001, jamanetwork.com/journals/jamapsychiatry/article-abstract/497958?redirect=true, 10.1001/archpsyc.1997.01830230033005.

Solzhenitsyn, Aleksandr. *Invisible Allies*. Washington, Counterpoint, 1997.

---. *The Oak and the Calf*. New York, Harper & Row, 1980.

Spijker, Jan, et al. "Duration of Major Depressive Episodes in the General Population: Results from the Netherlands Mental Health Survey and Incidence Study (NEMESIS)." *British Journal of Psychiatry*, vol. 181, no. 03, Sept. 2002, pp. 208–213, 10.1192/bjp.181.3.208.

Styron, William. *Darkness Visible: A Memoir of Madness*. New York, Random House, 1999.

"Suicide Statistics — AFSP." *AFSP*, 2018, afsp.org/about-suicide/suicide-statistics/.

Sullivan, P F, et al. "Genetic Epidemiology of Major Depression: Review and Meta-Analysis." *The American Journal of Psychiatry*, vol. 157, no. 10, Oct. 2000, pp. 1552–62, www.ncbi.nlm.nih.gov/pubmed/11007705, 10.1176/appi.ajp.157.10.1552.

Sullivan, Harry Stack, et al. *The Interpersonal Theory of Psychiatry*. New York; London, W. W. Norton & Company, 1968.

Tolstoy, Leo, translated by Aylmer Maude. *My Confession*. Digital Version. www.standardebooks.org/ebooks/leo-tolstoy/a-confession/aylmer-maude_louise-maude

Williams, Mark, et al. *The Mindful Way through Depression: Freeing Yourself from Chronic Unhappiness*. New York: London, The Guilford Press, 2007.

Notes

Preface

"nothing comes out of the blue…" O'Connor, Richard. *Undoing Depression*, Kindle Edition

Chapter 1

"9.5 percent of American adults…" NIMH, Any Mood Disorder Among Adults, www.nimh.nih.gov/health/statistics/prevalence/any-mood-disorder-among-adults.shtml

"one in every five Americans…" Cross-national comparisons of the prevalences and correlates of mental disorders, who.int/bulletin/archives/78(4)413.pdf

"two-thirds of all suicide…" DePaulo, Raymond, *Understanding Depression,* pp 132

"over thirty-one thousand…" Suicide Statistics — AFSP, afsp.org/about-suicide/suicide-statistics

"close to five hundred thousand…" Suicide across the world (2016), www.who.int/mental_health/prevention/suicide/suicideprevent/en/

"the bottom line…" O'Connor, Richard. *Undoing Depression*, Kindle Edition, Chapter 3, Subheading *A Distinction Without a Difference*

"to qualify for Major Depressive Disorder…" American Psychiatric Association, *DSM-4*, pp 327

"called a Major Depressive Episode…" American Psychiatric Association, *DSM-4*, pp 339

"To qualify for Dysthymic Disorder…" American Psychiatric Association, *DSM-4*, pp 349

"These three separate categories…" O'Connor, Richard. *Undoing Depression,* Kindle Edition, Chapter 3, Subheading *A Difference without Distinction*

"He cites a study…" O'Connor, Richard. *Undoing Depression,* Kindle Edition, Chapter 3, Subheading *A Difference without Distinction*

"major depressive episodes may occur during," American Psychiatric Association, *DSM-5*, pp 167

"scientifically meaningful differences," American Psychiatric Association, "Highlights of Changes from DSM-IV-TR to DSM-5," pp 4

"symptoms, family history, or treatment response," Black, Donald W, et al. *DSM-5 Guidebook,* pp 133

Chapter 2

Self-Descriptions of Depression

"Depressed people frequently describe..." for some good self-descriptions of depression, see Casey, Nell. *Unholy Ghost: Writers on Depression;* also see American Psychiatric Association, *DSM-5,* pp 163-164

Alienation from Sense of Self

"A phenomenon that a number..." Styron, William. *Darkness Visible,* pp 64

"From being a living person..." Casey, Nell. *Unholy Ghost: Writers on Depression,* from Essay *Walter Benjamin at the Dairy Queen,* by Larry McMurtry, pp 69

"I was acquiring a new..." Casey, Nell. *Unholy Ghost: Writers on Depression,* from Essay *Bodies in the Basement,* by Russell Banks, pp 35

"like living in a corpse..." Casey, Nell. *Unholy Ghost: Writers on Depression,* from Essay *A Better Place to Live,* by Maud Casey, pp 285

An Unstable Identity

"The struggle for identity is..." for good examples of this, see the brilliant essays in Casey, Nell. *Unholy Ghost: Writers on Depression*

Roots in Childhood

"Many say that there was a constant..." see essays in Casey, Nell. *Unholy Ghost: Writers on Depression*

External Blankness, Internal Strife

"One of the many things..." Casey, Nell. *Unholy Ghost: Writers on Depression,* from Essay *Planet No,* by Leslie Dormen, pp 236

Self-Hatred and Absence of Self-Esteem

"That they invariably exhibit low…" for the distinction between positive and negative self-esteem, see Brown, George W, et al. "Self-Esteem and Depression. 1. Measurement Issues and Prediction of Onset." Jul 1990.

Cognitive Biases

"prominent and pessimistic cognitive biases…" O'Connor, Richard. *Undoing Depression,* Kindle Edition, Chapter 8, Subheading *Distorted Perception and Bad Logic*

"they have a hard time remembering…" O'Connor, Richard. *Undoing Depression,* Kindle Edition, Chapter 2, Subheading *The Depressed Life*

"They tend to interpret…" Beck, Aaron and Brad Alford. *Depression: Causes and Treatment*, Chapter 10, Subheading *Typology of Cognitive Distortions*, pp 203-205

"Their view of the future…" Beck, Aaron and Brad Alford. *Depression: Causes and Treatment,* pp 24-25

"expects his misery will last forever…" Styron, William. *Darkness Visible*, pp 73

An Episodic Affliction

"About half of all depressive episodes… only a fourth last more than a year…" Spijker, Jan, et al. "Duration of Major Depressive Episodes in the General Population: Results from the Netherlands Mental Health Survey and Incidence Study (NEMESIS)." Sept 2002.

"about three percent last more than a decade…" is a conservative estimate from: Solomon, David A., et al. "Predicting Recovery from Episodes of Major Depression." Apr 2008.

"In at least 50 percent… and the more episodes of depression…" Williams, Mark, et al. *The Mindful Way through Depression*, Chapter 1, Subheading *When Unhappiness Turns into Depression . . . and Depression Won't Go Away,* pp 16

Course of the Illness

"bottoms out…" Beck, Aaron and Brad Alford. *Depression: Causes and Treatment,* pp 44 "a full psychological breakdown…" Solomon, Andrew. *Noonday Demon*, Chapter 2: Breakdowns

Immobile Depression and Workaholic Depression

"most people grow increasingly lethargic…" O'Connor, Richard. *Undoing Depression,* Kindle Edition, Chapter 7, Subheading *Can't-Get-Out-of-Bed Depression*

"spinning-your-wheels… really feel their depression…" O'Connor, Richard. *Undoing Depression*, Kindle Edition, Chapter 7, Subheading *Spinning-Your-Wheels Depression*

A Difference Between First and Subsequent Episodes

"An individual's very first episode… second episode… third and subsequent episodes…" Solomon, Andrew. *Noonday Demon*, pp 62-63; and O'Connor, Richard. *Undoing Depression,* Kindle Edition, Chapter 14, Subheading *Mindfulness-Based Therapy for Depression*

"this tragedy may be disguised…" Solomon, Andrew. *Noonday Demon*, pp 62

"out of the blue… by the person's own thought processes…" O'Connor, Richard. *Undoing Depression*, Kindle Edition, Chapter 20, Subheading *Nothing Comes Out of the Blue*; and Williams, Mark, et al. *The Mindful Way through Depression*, pp 17, 30

Avoiding their Feelings

"aversive relationships to their feelings…" O'Connor, Richard. Kindle Edition, Chapter 6: Emotions, First Section, No Subheading; and O'Connor, Richard. Kindle Edition, Chapter 4, Subheading *The Vicious Circle*; and Williams, Mark, et al. *The Mindful Way through Depression*, pp 119

"on some level… if she ever started crying…" Williams, Mark, et al. *The Mindful Way through Depression*, pp 134

The Vicious Circle

"vicious circle…" O'Connor, Richard. *Undoing Depression,* Kindle Edition, Chapter 4, Subheading *The Vicious Circle*

"for which they blame themselves even harder..." O'Connor, Richard. *Undoing Depression*, Kindle Edition, Chapter 1: Understanding Depression, First Section, No Subheading

"walk around with a vast hurt..." O'Connor, Richard. *Undoing Depression*, Kindle Edition

"ashamed of those very needs and desires..." O'Connor, Richard. *Undoing Depression*, Kindle Edition, Chapter 1: Understanding Depression, First Section, No Subheading

"the further they seek to withdraw into solitude..." O'Connor, Richard. *Undoing Depression*, Kindle Edition, Chapter 6, Subheading *Joy and Pride*

"appalls and drives away even those closest..." O'Connor, Richard. *Undoing Depression*, Kindle Edition, Chapter 14, Subheading *Family Support*; and DePaulo, Raymond, *Understanding Depression*, pp 128-131

"belief in the worst of all worlds..." O'Connor, Richard. *Undoing Depression*, Kindle Edition, Chapter 8, Subheading *Distorted Perceptions and Bad Logic*

"learned helplessness... which usually leads to actual failure..." O'Connor, Richard. *Undoing Depression*, Kindle Edition, Chapter 8, Subheading *Pessimism and Optimism*

"make major, life-ruining decisions..." O'Connor, Richard. *Undoing Depression*, Kindle Edition, Chapter 4, Subheading *The Vicious Circle*

"the symptoms of depression cause depression..." Solomon, Andrew. *Noonday Demon*, pp 61

Stress and Depression

"a close link between stress and depression..." a good review can be found in Monroe, Scott M., et al. "Major Life Events and Major Chronic Difficulties Are Differentially Associated with History of Major Depressive Episodes." Feb 2007.

"Stress is our body's so-called..." a good explanation of stress can be found in Sapolsky, Robert M. *Why Zebras Don't Get Ulcers*, Chapter 1

Stressors and Stabilizers

"intense stressor—such as divorce..." a good list of depression-causing events in Brown, George W, and Tirril O Harris. *Social Origins of Depression*, Kindle Edition. Table 2B. pp 104

"a major humiliation..." a good example of this type of event in Brown, George W. "Psychosocial Factors and Depression and Anxiety Disorders- Some Possible Implications for Biological Research." Jan 1996.

"genuine, ongoing life difficulties..." a list of these difficulties from Brown, George W, and Tirril O Harris. *Social Origins of Depression,* Kindle Edition, Chapter 8: Difficulties, pp 130-137; and Monroe, Scott M., et al. "Major Life Events and Major Chronic Difficulties Are Differentially Associated with History of Major Depressive Episodes." Feb 2007.

"about twice as likely..." Brown, George W, and Tirril O Harris. *Social Origins of Depression,* Kindle Edition, Chapter 8: Difficulties, pp 138

"long-term stressors..." Hari, Johann. *Lost Connections,* pp 50

"help them diffuse, cope with, or resolve..." a good description of factors that mitigate depression in Sapolsky, Robert M. *Why Zebras Don't Get Ulcers,* Chapter 13

"external stabilizers that shield against depression include..." Brown, George W, and Tirril O Harris. *Social Origins of Depression,* Kindle Edition, Chapter 11: Vulnerability, pp 173-191

"the internal stabilizer include... self-esteem backing those skills..." Brown, George W, and Tirril O Harris. *Social Origins of Depression,* Kindle Edition, Chapter 15: Depression and Loss, pp 235 ("a sense of one's ability to control the world and thus repair damage") and pp 247 ("the overlap between outer and inner resources"); and for how negative self-esteem increases vulnerability to depression, see Brown, George W, et al. "Social Support, Self-Esteem and Depression." Nov 1986, and Brown, George W, et al. "Self-Esteem and Depression. 1. Measurement Issues and Prediction of Onset." Jul 1990; and for how positive self-esteem protects against depression, see Brown, George W. "Self-Esteem and Depression. III. Aetiological Issues." Oct 1990.

"a 'good enough' marriage" Solomon, Andrew. *Noonday Demon*, pp 63

Vulnerable Demographics

"Women, at least across Western societies..." Solomon, Andrew. *Noonday Demon*, pp 175

"The elderly living in nursing homes…" Solomon, Andrew. *Noonday Demon*, pp 528

The poor have two to three…" Solomon, Andrew. *Noonday Demon*, pp 336

"And gay men…" Solomon, Andrew. *Noonday Demon*, pp 202, and Cochran, Susan D, et al. "Prevalence of Mental Disorders, Psychological Distress, and Mental Health Services Use among Lesbian, Gay, and Bisexual Adults in the United States." Feb 2003.

Adverse Childhood Experiences

"physical abuse… sexual abuse… emotional abuse… battered mother… household substance abuse… mental illness in household… criminal household member" the list of adverse childhood experience in Chapman, Daniel P., et al. "Adverse Childhood Experiences and the Risk of Depressive Disorders in Adulthood." Oct 2004

"neglect…" as an adverse childhood experience included in Cheong, E Von, et al. "Adverse Childhood Experiences (ACEs) and Later-Life Depression: Perceived Social Support as a Potential Protective Factor." Sept 2017; and Brown, George W. "Psychosocial Factors and Depression and Anxiety Disorders- Some Possible Implications for Biological Research." Jan 1996.

"parents' deaths, or… a parent's suicide…" Berg, Lisa, et al. "Parental Death during Childhood and Depression in Young Adults - a National Cohort Study." Apr 2016.

"by emotional abuse toward females…" Chapman, Daniel P., et al. "Adverse Childhood Experiences and the Risk of Depressive Disorders in Adulthood." Oct 2004.

"being the child of a depressed parent…" Solomon, Andrew. *Noonday Demon*, pp 181

"living through the suicide of a parent…" Berg, Lisa, et al. "Parental Death during Childhood and Depression in Young Adults - a National Cohort Study." Apr 2016.

"Each additional ACE substantially increases…" all stats are from Chapman, Daniel P., et al. "Adverse Childhood Experiences and the Risk of Depressive Disorders in Adulthood." Oct 2004.

"the earlier in a child's life they occur…" for parental death and suicide in Berg, Lisa, et al. "Parental Death during Childhood and Depression in Young Adults - a National Cohort Study." Apr 2016; and for many others in Schalinski, Inga, et al. "Type and Timing of Adverse Childhood Experiences Differentially Affect

Severity of PTSD, Dissociative and Depressive Symptoms in Adult Inpatients."
Aug 2016.

"It has now been established…" Solomon, Andrew. *Noonday Demon*, pp 187

"children as young as two or three…" Solomon, Andrew. *Noonday Demon*, pp 181

"remain much more susceptible… tend to be much more intense…" Beck, Aaron
and Brad Alford. *Depression: Causes and Treatment*, pp 196-197

The Compound Effect of Stressors

"In one landmark study of adult women…" Brown, George W, and Tirril O
Harris. *Social Origins of Depression*, Kindle Edition, Chapter 11: Vulnerability, pp 181

Anxiety and Other Mental Disorders

"also affect anxiety reactivity…" Sapolsky, Robert M. *Why Zebras Don't Get Ulcers*,
Chapters 15-16

"51 to 68 percent of people…" O'Connor, Richard. *Undoing Depression*, Kindle
Edition, Chapter 3, Subheading *Depression, Anxiety, and Stress*; and Chapter 13,
Subheading *Depression and Anxiety*

"in 62 percent of all cases…" Kessler, Ronald C. "Lifetime and 12-Month
Prevalence of DSM-III-R Psychiatric Disorders in the United States." Jan 1994,
cited in O'Connor, Richard. *Undoing Depression*, Kindle Edition, Chapter 13,
Subheading *Depression and Anxiety*

Genes and Depression

"Depression often runs in the family…" a good summary can be found in
DePaulo, Raymond, *Understanding Depression*, Chapter 7: Genes and Depression:
The Fateful Inheritance, pp 88-90

"If one identical twin… if a fraternal twin…" Beck, Aaron and Brad Alford.
Depression: Causes and Treatment, pp 142-143

"the overall pattern remains the same…" a good summary can be found in
Hammen, Constance. *Depression*, pp 61-62

"Scientists have discovered one crucial gene…" Caspi, A. "Influence of Life Stress
on Depression: Moderation by a Polymorphism in the 5-HTT Gene." Jul 2003.

"at around 38 percent..." Sullivan, P F, et al. "Genetic Epidemiology of Major Depression: Review and Meta-Analysis." Oct. 2000; and Kendler, Kenneth S, et al. "A Swedish National Twin Study of Lifetime Major Depression." Jan 2006; both cited in Beck, Aaron and Brad Alford. *Depression: Causes and Treatment*, pp 143

Unrecognized Depression

"I knew something was wrong..." Casey, Nell. *Unholy Ghost: Writers on Depression*, from Essay *Fading to Gray*, by Lee Stringer, pp 113

"like many postpartum depressions..." for great examples of this, see Karraa, Walker. *Transformed by Postpartum Depression*, Chapter 3

Bipolar Depression

"replaced with its exact opposite: mania..." a good summary in DePaulo, Raymond, *Understanding Depression*, Chapter 2: The Experience of Mania: Bipolar Disorder

Additional Symptoms

"extremely sensitive to rejection... overly concerned with other people's opinion..." O'Connor, Richard. *Undoing Depression*, Kindle Edition, Chapter 10, Subheading *Rejection Sensitivity*

"lose the ability to find humor..." Beck, Aaron and Brad Alford. *Depression: Causes and Treatment*, pp 22

"sometimes harbor great anger..." O'Connor, Richard. *Undoing Depression*, Kindle Edition, Chapter 5: The World of Depression, First Section, No Subheading

"diminished sex drive, impotence, or an inability to orgasm..." Beck, Aaron and Brad Alford. *Depression: Causes and Treatment*, pp 34-35

Chapter 3

"Let us make no bones..." Solomon, Andrew. *Noonday Demon*, pp 29

"hinges on the elimination of theory..." Greenberg, Gary. *Manufacturing Depression*, pp 252

"a biopsychosocial perspective..." Hari, Johann. *Lost Connections*, pp 54

"Adverse childhood experiences..." Hari, Johann. *Lost Connections*, Chapter 4

"rejection by a real or potential lover… diagnosis of serious illness…" Beck, Aaron and Brad Alford. *Depression: Causes and Treatment*, pp 249

"the death of a loved one," American Psychiatric Association, *DSM-4*, pp 342

"involvement in an abusive, dependent, or jealous relationship…" O'Connor, Richard. *Undoing Perpetual Stress*, pp 397-400

"living a lonelily, isolated lifestyle…" Hari, Johann. *Lost Connections,* Chapter 7

"getting addicted to drugs, gambling, or alcohol…" DePaulo, Raymond, *Understanding Depression,* Chapter 10

Chapter 4:

"we have made but small advances…" Solomon, Andrew. *Noonday Demon*, pp 171

"somewhat better than a placebo… 30 to 40 percent of cases…" O'Connor, Richard. *Undoing Depression,* Kindle Edition, Chapter 13, Subheading *The Dark Side of Medication*

"If one pharmaceutical fails to work…" DePaulo, Raymond, *Understanding Depression,* Chapter 14

"the biggest and most thorough study…" National Institute of Mental Health. "NIMH» Questions and Answers about the NIMH Sequenced Treatment Alternatives to Relieve Depression (STAR*D) Study — All Medication Levels." Nov 2006.

"give the example of General Tecumseh Sherman…" O'Connor, Richard. *Undoing Depression,* Kindle Edition, Chapter 6, Subheading *Anger*

"John Stuart Mill, who's autobiography…" Mill, John Stuart. *The Autobiography of John Stuart Mill,* Chapter 5.

"almost every night I fully expected…" Solzhenitsyn, Aleksandr. *The Oak and the Calf,* pp 103-104

"one Cambodian farmer who lost…" Hari, Johann. *Lost Connections,* pp 14

"the dodo bird effect…" Greenberg, Gary. *Manufacturing Depression,* pp 300-301

"intelligence and insight… type of insight… are really secondary…" Solomon, Andrew. *Noonday Demon*, pp 111

"therapy alone is about as effective as antidepressants alone… around 80 percent of patients…" *Noonday Demon*, pp 104

"allows a person to make sense..." Solomon, Andrew. *Noonday Demon*, pp 104

"A full course of treatment... over 75 percent of the time..." Solomon, Andrew. *Noonday Demon*, pp 121

"return to the same comfortable..." O'Connor, Richard. *Undoing Depression,* Kindle Edition

"a peculiar assortment of conditions..." Solomon, Andrew. *Noonday Demon*, pp 402

Chapter 5

"inability to feel... a big heavy blanket that..." O'Connor, Richard. *Undoing Depression,* Kindle Edition

"sadness as you had known it..." Solomon, Andrew. *Noonday Demon*, pp 16

"We know from Freud..." this was one of the earliest insights guiding Freud's work, already described (in 1895) in Freud, Sigmund, and Josef Breuer. *Studies on Hysteria*

Chapter 6

"aren't a relic of the beloved person... but the various ways..." a great example of this can be found in Epstein, Seymour. *Cognitive Experiential Theory*, pp 219

"Drug or alcohol is present in roughly 18 percent..." Kessler, R C, et al. "Comorbidity of DSM-III-R Major Depressive Disorder in the General Population: Results from the US National Comorbidity Survey." Jun 1996.

"psychosis is present in roughly 14 percent..." Johnson, J, et al. "The Validity of Major Depression with Psychotic Features Based on a Community Study." Dec 1991.

"gets much more complicated... prognosis becomes much bleaker..." O'Connor, Richard. *Undoing Depression,* Kindle Edition, Chapter 7, Subheading *Depression, Alcohol, and Drugs*, and Chapter 3, Subheading *Major Depression with Psychotic Features*; and also in DePaulo, Raymond, *Understanding Depression,* Chapter 10, Subheading *How Drugs and Alcohol Affect Treatment,* pp 124-125

Chapter 8

"Abraham Maslow observed that these relationships..." see Maslow, Abraham. *Toward a Psychology of Being*, Chapter 3: Deficiency and Growth Motivation; and Maslow, Abraham. *Motivation and Personality*, Chapter 12: Love in Self-Actualizing People

"the adolescent girl needs admiration…" Maslow, Abraham. *Toward a Psychology of Being*, pp 36

"when nothing seems worth the effort…" Rand, Ayn. *Atlas Shrugged*, pp 711

"deep and enduring feeling of sadness…" Epstein, Seymour. *Cognitive Experiential Theory*, pp 209

"the refusal of grief…" Butler, Judith. *The Psychic Life of Power Theories in Subjection*, pp 142; cited in Epstein, Seymour. *Cognitive Experiential Theory*, pp 213

"incomplete mourning…" Bowlby, John. *Attachment and Loss. Vol. 3 Loss, Sadness and Depression*; cited in Epstein, Seymour. *Cognitive Experiential Theory*, pp 213

"Freud conceived this mechanism of repression…" Freud, Sigmund. *Freud Complete Works*. Freud calls the superego "the representative for us of every moral restriction," which "goes back to the influence of parents, educators, and so on" (pp 4676). Freud says the superego "represents the claims of morality" and that "our moral sense of guilt is the expression of the tension between the ego and the superego" (pp 4669). Freud calls the superego (at this point called the "ego ideal") our "chief influence in repression" (pp 3801). Freud says that the superego "makes itself noisily heard" in "the form of reproaches" (pp 4529). Freud says the "conscience"—the faculty that objects to certain deeds a person commits by punishing him with "distressing reproaches"—is "independent" from the superego, but is "one of its functions" (pp 4668).

"Man's reason is his moral faculty…" Rand, Ayn. *Atlas Shrugged*, pp 931

"became widely accepted among Freudian psychologists…" O'Connor, Richard. *Undoing Depression*, Kindle Edition, Chapter 3: Diagnosing Depression, First Section, No Subheading; a good history of this can be found in Rei, Herbert E. *Depression in Childhood: A Survey of Some Pertinent Contributions*. 1996

"the kids of abusive parents… commonly blame that abuse on themselves…" Epstein, Seymour. *Cognitive Experiential Theory*, pp 213

"Other writers on depression affirmed this…" it was initially stated by Harry Stack Sullivan, see Sullivan, Harry Stack, et al. *The Interpersonal Theory of Psychiatry*; and was recently echoed in Hari, Johann. *Lost Connections*, pp 114

"Richard O'Connor was right in viewing repression…" O'Connor, Richard. *Undoing Depression*, Kindle Edition, Chapter 2, Subheading *Depressed Emotional Skills*

"a loss of what seems to the patient…" Arieti, Silvano, and Jules Bemporad. *Severe and Mild Depression*, Digital Edition, pp 387

"one of the chief risks of divorce…" O'Connor, Richard. *Undoing Depression,* Kindle Edition

"often internalize blame…" Solomon, Andrew. *Noonday Demon,* pp 257; some good corroboration and examples of this can be found in Bowlby, John. *Attachment and Loss. Vol. 3 Loss, Sadness and Depression,* pp 382-389

"An American soldier in the Korean war…" Beck, Aaron, and Sigmund Valin. "Psychotic Depressive Reactions in Soldiers Who Accidentally Killed Their Buddies." Nov 1953; partially reproduced in Beck, Aaron and Brad Alford. *Depression: Causes and Treatment,* pp 85-87

"best friend [and] soulmate… You killed the one you…" Samman, Josh. *The Housekeeper,* pp 211, 216

"there are also depressions without feelings of worthlessness…" Epstein, Seymour. *Cognitive Experiential Theory,* pp 210

Chapter 10

"about 10 to 20 percent of all cases…" is an estimate based on the 12-month prevalence rate of bipolar disorder (1.8% according to American Psychiatric Association. *DSM-5,* pp 136) and unipolar depression (which we know to be about 9.5%, according to NIMH, Any Mood Disorder Among Adults, www.nimh.nih.gov/health/statistics/prevalence/any-mood-disorder-among-adults.shtml)

"Mania is exuberance gone amok…" Jamison, Kay R. *Exuberance: The Passion for Life,* pp 100
"the common pitfalls of mania include…" DePaulo, Raymond, *Understanding Depression,* Chapter 2: The Experience of Mania: Bipolar Disorder

"John Bowlby showed this to be a fairly common…" Bowlby, John. *Attachment and Loss. Vol. 3 Loss, Sadness and Depression,* pp 146-147

"The depressed person thinks his depression is permanent…" Beck, Aaron and Brad Alford. *Depression: Causes and Treatment,* pp 230

Chapter 11

"depression is a chronic disease that…" O'Connor, Richard. *Undoing Depression,* Kindle Edition

"a person who's had one Major Depressive Episode, has… a 50 percent chance… a 70 percent chance… a 90 percent change… almost 100 percent guaranteed…" Beck, Aaron and Brad Alford. *Depression: Causes and Treatment,* pp 62

"some stress pushes us over…" O'Connor, Richard. *Undoing Depression,* Kindle Edition

"a low-grade dysthymia always there…" O'Connor, Richard. *Undoing Depression,* Kindle Edition

"the next episodes tend to be…" that they are "shorter" is from Spijker, Jan, et al. "Duration of Major Depressive Episodes in the General Population: Results from the Netherlands Mental Health Survey and Incidence Study (NEMESIS)." Sept 2002.; that they are "closer together" is from Beck, Aaron and Brad Alford. *Depression: Causes and Treatment,* pp 62; and they are "more intense" is from Maj, M, et al. "Pattern of Recurrence of Illness after Recovery from an Episode of Major Depression: A Prospective Study." Jun 1992.

"The best predictor of whether a person's depression will become recurrent…" O'Connor, Richard. *Undoing Depression,* Kindle Edition, Chapter 3, Subheading *Depression, Anxiety, and Stress*

Chapter 12

"'constellation' of 'interrelated negative attitudes'…" Beck, Aaron and Brad Alford. *Depression: Causes and Treatment,* pp 247

"skills of depression…" O'Connor, Richard. *Undoing Depression,* Kindle Edition, Chapter 2, Subheading *The Depressed Life*

"predepressive constellation…" Beck, Aaron and Brad Alford. *Depression: Causes and Treatment,* pp 247

"skills of depression… thinking feeling and doing… a big, intertwined ball of string…" O'Connor, Richard. *Undoing Depression,* Kindle Edition, Chapter 2, Subheading *The Depressed Life*

"I am not my thoughts…" Segal, Zindel V, et al. *Mindfulness-Based Cognitive Therapy for Depression (Second Edition),* pp 413

"appearances in conscious…" is an excellent descriptive phrase from another good book on mindfulness: Harris, Sam. *Waking Up,* pp 87

"During periods of recovery, a chronic depressive's worldview…" Segal, Zindel V, et al. *Mindfulness-Based Cognitive Therapy for Depression (Second Edition),* pp 27

"lack[s] confidence in [his] own judgment…" O'Connor, Richard. *Undoing Depression,* Kindle Edition "his habitual depressive beliefs... it's those that he now thinks are true..." Segal, Zindel V, et al. *Mindfulness-Based Cognitive Therapy for Depression (Second Edition),* pp 27-29

"to notice when he's beginning to ruminate... interrupting the positive feedback..." O'Connor, Richard. *Undoing Depression,* Kindle Edition, Chapter 14, Subheading *Mindfulness-Based Therapy for Depression*
"It hasn't, however, shown any effectiveness in patients..." Ma, S Helen, and John D Teasdale. "Mindfulness-Based Cognitive Therapy for Depression: Replication and Exploration of Differential Relapse Prevention Effects." Feb 2004.

"I am my own judge, jury..." Beck, Aaron, and Sigmund Valin. "Psychotic Depressive Reactions in Soldiers Who Accidentally Killed Their Buddies." Nov 1953.

"a bad habit we had..." After Girlfriend's Death, Josh Samman Takes Guilt, Grief into UFC 181. mmajunkie.com/2014/12/after-girlfriends-death-josh-samman-takes-guilt-grief-into-ufc-181. Accessed May 2019

"indistinguishable from depression... the bereavement exclusion..." Greenberg, Gary. *Manufacturing Depression,* pp 246-247

"a normal reaction to the death... significant loss[es]... financial ruin, losses from..." American Psychiatric Association. *DSM-5,* pp 161, 716-717

"All my happiness was..." Mill, John Stuart. *The Autobiography of John Stuart Mill,* Chapter 5

"In John Stuart Mill's case, the loss..." Mill, John Stuart. *The Autobiography of John Stuart Mill,* Chapter 5

"Aleksandr Solzhenitsyn escaped his depression..." Solzhenitsyn, Aleksandr. *Invisible Allies,* pp 54

Chapter 13

"the frustration of so many impulses..." Lewis, C S. *A Grief Observed,* pp 23

Chapter 14

"Rhesus monkeys briefly separated from..." Harlow, Harry F., and Stephen J. Suomi. "Induced Depression in Monkeys." Nov 1974; and O'Connor, Richard. *Undoing Depression,* Kindle Edition, Chapter 17, Subheading *Monkey Depression*

"Male baboons, for example, will..." all information on baboon dominance from Kummer, Hans. *In Quest of The Sacred Baboon,* pp 34, 212, and 283; and Sapolsky, Robert M. *A Primate's Memoir,* pp 234

"self concept… may be the evolutionary primordium…" Price, John, et al. "The Social Competition Hypothesis of Depression." Mar 1994.

"The overthrown alpha baboons…" Kummer, Hans. *In Quest of The Sacred Baboon*, pp 237

"A dominant lobster defeated ins…" Peterson, Jordan B. *12 Rules for Life*, pp 6-7

"constellation of changes…" Sapolsky, Robert M. *A Primate's Memoir*, pp 177

"Jordan Peterson makes a highly compelling case…" Peterson, Jordan B. *12 Rules for Life*, pp 16-17

"Giving a lobster Prozac…" Peterson, Jordan B. *12 Rules for Life*, pp 7

Chapter 15

"Richard O'Connor draws an important distinction…" O'Connor, Richard. *Undoing Depression*, Kindle Edition, Chapter 14: Psychotherapy, Self-Help, and Other Means to Recovery. First Section, No Subheading

"And ketamine… with success rates that blow antidepressants…" for history and effectiveness of ketamine, see Greenberg, Gary. *Manufacturing Depression*, pp 174-177; and "Erowid Ketamine Vault." www.erowid.org/chemicals/ketamine. Accessed May 2019.

"psilocybin can generate ecstatic, acutely pleasurable…" Griffiths, R. R., et al. "Psilocybin Can Occasion Mystical-Type Experiences Having Substantial and Sustained Personal Meaning and Spiritual Significance;" and Maslow, Abraham. *Religions, Values, and Peak Experiences*, Appendix A and Appendix D

"its efficacy as a treatment… much higher than antidepressants…" Carhart-Harris, Robin L, et al. "Psilocybin with Psychological Support for Treatment-Resistant Depression: An Open-Label Feasibility Study." Jul 2016; cited in Pollan, Michael. *How to Change Your Mind*, pp 376

"bad trips can be easily avoided…" Pollan, Michael. *How to Change Your Mind*, pp 14-15

"can actually prove fatal…" for more information on the interactions between antidepressants and psychedelics, see Bonson, Kit. *Info on Hallucinogens with Antidepressants*. erowid.org/chemicals/maois/maois_info4.shtml. Accessed May 2019.

Made in the USA
Middletown, DE
27 September 2019